Praise for *Yoga for Meditators*

"I am sure Charlotte Bell's jewel of a book will become a classic for meditators. Whether new to the practice or a longtime practitioner, readers will learn quick, simple, and practical solutions for finding ease in sitting. What shines through in this book is the balance of compassionately tending to (and in many cases preventing) the common aches and pains that can arise in meditation with the genuine practice of mindfulness."

—Donna Farhi, author of *Teaching Yoga*

"*Yoga for Meditators* is friendly, clear, and full of the wisdom of experience, just like its author, my friend, Charlotte Bell, longtime meditator and experienced yoga practitioner. I cannot think of a better book to recommend to anyone wanting to sit with ease on the cushion. Charlotte offers the reader the comfort of her warmth and knowledge, and it is a much needed and welcome gift. Highly recommended for all levels of practitioners."

—Judith Hanson Lasater, Ph.D., P.T., coauthor of *What We Say Matters*

"*Yoga for Meditators* is an invaluable support for any practitioner who meets the inevitable discomforts of sitting still for long periods of time. Charlotte's book is a comprehensive guide to achieving a well-balanced posture that serves as a foundation for a mind of calmness. The instructions for the postures are accessible for all, including those who have never ventured into the discipline of yoga. I highly recommend this book."

—Christina Feldman, author of *Compassion: Listening to the Cries of the World*

"Finally, a book in an easy-to-understand format for today's yoga students and teachers that will illuminate and support their meditation practice. I love this book and will recommend it on my website and in teacher trainings."

—Jenny Otto, Body Balance Certification Program and Trainings

"This is an extremely useful book. I wish I had had it when I began my meditation practice and will recommend it to my students. It is patient, kind, intelligent, and down to earth. It is a great pleasure to read this book for its valuable teaching and also to spend some time with this wonderful teacher."
—Daniel Doen Silberberg, Sensei, author of *Wonderland: The Zen of Alice*

"In an age when yoga has become a fitness fad, *Yoga for Meditators* provides a much-needed glimpse into the deeper dimensions of yogic practice. Without imposing any doctrine, this book provides real and practical aids to add a spiritual dimension for the yoga practitioner and an honored place for the body in any meditative practice. A must-read for those serious about the interior life."
—The Reverend Michael Mayor, Episcopal Priest and Spiritual Director of All Saints Episcopal Church, Salt Lake City

"In *Yoga for Meditators*, Charlotte Bell gives simple, concise, and useful information to help readers with their meditation practice. Even for first-time meditators, her teaching will guide your body to be comfortable and your mind to quiet."
—Cora Wen, founder of Yoga Bloom, Cupertino, CA

"This book is what has been missing from all the how-to books out there on yoga. Charlotte not only tells us how to practice specific poses, but also reminds us why we practice them in the first place. A wonderful how-to-take-it-to-the-next-level yoga book that you will definitely want in your library. You *can* feel comfortable while sitting in meditation; this book gives you the map to get there."
—D'ana Baptiste, founder of Centered City Yoga, Salt Lake City

Yoga for Meditators

Rodmell Press Yoga Shorts

By Charlotte Bell
Yoga For Meditators

By Sandy Blaine
Yoga for Computer Users
Yoga for Healthy Knees

By Shoosh Lettick Crotzer
Yoga for Fibromyalgia

By Judith Hanson Lasater, Ph.D., P.T.
Yoga Abs
Yoga for Pregnancy

rodmell press

YOGA SHORTS

YOGA

FOR MEDITATORS

POSES TO SUPPORT YOUR SITTING PRACTICE

▼　　▼　　▼　　▼　　▼　　▼　　▼　　▼

Charlotte Bell

RODMELL PRESS　　　BERKELEY, CALIFORNIA, 2012

Library of Congress Cataloging-in-Publication Data

Bell, Charlotte, 1955-
Yoga for meditators : poses to support your sitting practice
/ Charlotte Bell.
p. cm. — (Rodmell press yoga shorts)
Includes index.
ISBN 978-1-930485-30-3 (pbk. : alk. paper)
1. Yoga. 2. Sitting position. I. Title.
B132.Y6B4228 2012
613.7'046—dc23

2011046368

Printed and bound in China
First edition

ISBN-13: 978-1-930485-30-3
16 15 14 13 12   1 2 3 4 5 6 7 8 9 10

Editors: Holly Hammond, Linda Cogozzo
Design: Gopa & Ted2, Inc.
Indexer: Ty Koontz
Asana Illustrations: Sharon Ellis
Anatomy Illustration: Lauren Keswick
Author Photo: Roz Newmark
Lithographer: Kwong Fat Offset Printing Co., Ltd.

Distributed by Publishers Group West

Contents

▼ ▼ ▼ ▼ ▼ ▼ ▼

Acknowledgments

▼ ▼ ▼ ▼ ▼ ▼ ▼ ▼ ▼ ▼ ▼

I've been exploring the intersection between yoga asana and meditation since the mid-1980s. So when Linda Cogozzo suggested the idea of this book to me, it immediately felt like a perfect fit. I'm forever grateful for Linda's insight and support. So, first and foremost, thanks to Linda and to Donald Moyer, copublishers at Rodmell Press, for offering me the opportunity to share these ideas that are so precious to me.

This book would not be possible had I not had the good fortune to explore practice with so many wise and insightful teachers. To my meditation and yoga teachers, Pujari and Abhilasha, I am infinitely grateful for your unconditional love and support for so many years. Every trip to their Last Resort Retreat Center has been a life-changing experience. Thanks also to Christina Feldman, Daniel Silberberg, Joseph Goldstein, and Reverend Michael Mayor.

In the realm of yoga asana, I'm grateful to the many wise teachers with whom I've had the opportunity to study. These six mentors and friends have been especially inspiring: Donna Farhi, Judith Hanson Lasater, Elise Miller, Jenny Otto, B.K.S. Iyengar, and the late Mary Dunn. Special thanks to Donna for teaching me about the dynamic relationship between breath and asana, and for teaching me how to live in partnership with gravity. Without these two insights, my asana and meditation practices would be far less graceful.

I wish to express immeasurable gratitude to my longtime teaching colleagues and dharma friends in Salt Lake City: Roz Newmark, Marlena Lambert, Lorie Nielson, Kathy Lung, Heidi O'Donoghue, Joan Degiorgio, Erin Geesaman-Rabke, Yael Calhoun, Jacqueline Morasco, Mary Johnston-Coursey, Lin Ostler, and Jay Jones. Additionally, many thanks to Roz for shooting the photos that served as resource material for the wonderful illustrations in this book.

Thanks also to my Red Rock Rondo cohorts for allowing me to practice musical meditation every time we play together: Phillip Bimstein, Hal Cannon, Harold Carr, Flavia Cervino-Wood, and Kate MacLeod. Warm, fuzzy thanks to my feline friends, Jazzy, Pushkin, and Lily, who took turns camping out in my lap and spiced up my typing during their occasional traverses across the keyboard.

I'm ever grateful to Phillip Bimstein for his love and encouragement, and for reading my manuscript with eyes far fresher than mine could be. And thanks to my birth family, the late Bob and Mary Jane Bell, and my sisters, Martha and Anne, for their great talent, heart, and unique sense of humor.

Finally, I'm grateful to all my students over these many years for their support, insight, humor, and inspiration. You have given far more than you can imagine.

Introduction

▼ ▼ ▼ ▼ ▼ ▼ ▼ ▼ ▼ ▼ ▼

"YOGA IS THE SETTLING of the mind into silence." Silence. Like the deafening stillness of a million-starred night in the desert. Like a lake on a windless day, so clear you can see through to the tiniest stone resting on its floor. Like the sky, undisturbed by the rains, snows, winds, and clouds that temporarily obscure its infinite nature. Like the pause between two breaths. Silence.

According to Sanskrit scholar Alistair Shearer's translation of *The Yoga Sutras of Patanjali* (New York: Harmony / Bell Tower, 2002), "the settling of the mind into silence" is the very definition of the ancient art of yoga. This defining aphorism is the second of 196 verses that make up this comprehensive text. All the other sutras serve to flesh out the meaning of this verse and provide a framework for its practice.

The framework provided by the sutras is called the Eight Limbs of Yoga. It includes *yama* (five moral precepts), *niyama* (daily practices), *asana* (poses), *pranayama* (breathing practices), *pratyahara* (retirement of the senses), *dharana* (concentration), *dhyana* (meditation), and *samadhi* (the completely settled mind). The last three of these are considered to be the heart of yoga, and distinctions between them are subtle. Each contains elements of the others. Each embodies, in its own way, a mind settling into silence.

Way back in 1988, in my seventh year of yoga practice, I decided to explore the silence of meditation for myself. As a committed yoga student, I'd heard that yoga was really more about meditation than about poses, but up until then I didn't feel a need to look into meditation. The lovely sense of peace I felt after my daily yoga practice was satisfying enough.

In the summer of 1986, I attended a yoga retreat at the Last Resort Retreat Center in southern Utah. There I dipped a tentative toe into the waters of meditation. Three times each day for a week, our intimate group of eight students and two teachers sat in a circle on hardwood benches with the intention of collecting our minds onto the experience of breathing. I found these sessions to be mostly pleasant and sometimes even energizing—my wandering mind notwithstanding. We spent one entire day in silence. I left the retreat feeling a profound sense of quiet and ease.

So in 1988, when I decided to dive headlong into meditation and embark on my first five-day, silent vipassana meditation retreat, I thought I had at least an idea of what it might be like. However, it would not be an exaggeration to say that during the first two days, sitting long hours in meditation was the most challenging and humbling endeavor I'd ever attempted. My mind behaved like the proverbial wild monkey, leaping from one embarrassing obsession or banal melody to the next with amazing agility.

But I somewhat expected this; I'd sat in meditation with my endlessly wandering mind eighteen months before. However, the physical discomfort I felt took me completely by surprise. Sitting three times a day at a yoga retreat did not prepare me for sitting seven hours a day in forty-five-minute to one-hour sessions. At some point, every part of my body chimed in, and sometimes shouted at me, pummeling me with its resistance. My knees screamed, my back and shoulders veritably shrieked. None of this helped my attitude, which became more dour with each agonizing minute.

But help was on the way. Unlike most vipassana meditation retreats back in those times, the Last Resort's schedule had a built-in body rescue plan. The teachers, Pujari and Abhilasha Keays, had studied yoga extensively in India with B.K.S. Iyengar. Each day's schedule had a yoga break, a delicious hour-long asana session designed to calm and energize, and to work out accumulated tensions in the body. Over the years, these sessions saved many a meditator at the Last Resort from becoming overwhelmed by physical discomfort.

Physical discomfort is not a product of the sitting itself. Rather, discomfort arises because in meditation we endeavor to sit still without moving. In daily life circumstances, when we sit for long periods of time, we automatically and unconsciously adjust ourselves to avoid pain as it arises. As far as the body is concerned, sitting on a meditation bench or *zafu* (meditation cushion) for seven or eight hours is really not a whole lot different from sitting at a computer for the same amount of time—except that when we're sitting at a computer, we constantly move and adjust, and most of our attention is focused on the screen in front of us instead of on what's happening in our body and mind. When we're sitting in meditation, we're mindful of every last stabbing, burning, straining, vibrating, itching, or pulling sensation, and because we're focused on it, it often feels like an assault.

The ancient yogis recognized this, and over millennia the practice of asana, the third of the Eight Limbs, was developed and refined to alleviate the physical rigors of sitting practice. Asana, the practice of physical postures, was specifically intended to relax the body and calm the nervous system, giving the mind a supportive environment in which to find stillness.

Traditional asana practice, as described in the Hatha Yoga Pradipika, the traditional text that outlines hatha yoga practice, focuses mostly on breathing practices and seated poses. The more athletic and physically challenging poses came to yoga through Western gymnastics, introduced to Indian yogis during the years the British Empire colonized the country.

Asana practice, by its very nature, is about preparing the body for meditation. So a book on yoga for meditators may seem redundant. All yoga is for meditators, after all. Still, there are poses that I have found to be optimal in addressing the specific physical challenges that arise during meditation, and it is in this spirit that I offer the practices in this book.

How to Use This Book

The book has four parts. In part 1, "Taking a Seat: Steady and Comfortable," you will find suggestions that address the most common physical issues that can cause discomfort during sitting. Part 2, "Yoga Poses for Sitting Meditation," presents asanas to guide you to a more easeful practice. Whether you practice vipassana, Zen, Transcendental, kriya, or any other kind of sitting meditation, these poses will help you collect the mind, awaken the spine, relax the base, soften the shoulders, and quiet the body-mind. In part 3, "Practicing Yoga," I suggest asana sequences, but I encourage you to mix and match poses to create sequences that suit your unique needs. Practicing even a single pose before or after meditation is beneficial. In part 4, "Alternate Meditation Postures," I discuss the other three traditional meditation postures—walking, standing, and lying down—and offer suggestions for creating ease in each.

The silent, peaceful mind is our birthright; it lives inside us all. Our minds and bodies are interwoven. When the body is at ease, the mind has a much easier time settling into silence. May your asana and meditation practices uncover the peace that already lives within.

Part 1:

Taking a Seat: Steady and Comfortable

▼   ▼   ▼   ▼   ▼   ▼   ▼   ▼   ▼   ▼   ▼   ▼

Setting Up: Finding the Right Support

DURING A QUESTION-AND-ANSWER session on a meditation retreat I led many years ago, one participant asked, "Why do we have to sit in such an uncomfortable position?" I knew what she meant. After years of sitting on a bench or cushion with no back support—with aching knees, low back, and shoulders—I had often wondered the same thing.

I pondered her question for a few moments, and then the answer came: Any position you sit in for a long period of time is going to get uncomfortable after a while. Whether you're sitting on a hard wooden bench with no back support or luxuriating in the most ergonomically supportive lounger, after a while your body is going to want to move.

Perhaps this sitting meditation scenario is familiar to you: You've been sitting a little while, and you suddenly notice that you're slumping a bit. You immediately correct by jerking your body back to a more upright position. Not long after, you notice you're slumping again, and once again you correct your position. The cycle can happen over and over in the course of a sitting. This little dance could be a sign that the spine is out of congruence, that your basic sitting position is not self-sustaining.

Traditional sitting postures—whether on a bench, zafu, or some other type of support—were developed to make the most of the body's natural energy flow. An upright, neutrally aligned spine allows for the most efficient movement of energy. When the spine, and therefore the spinal cord, is in an easy, neutral position, the nervous system has a much better chance of finding equilibrium, which creates a supportive environment for the mind to quiet.

When the spine is out of integrity, we struggle. Struggle creates an uncomfortable combination of agitation and fatigue. As we spend muscular energy to support the spine in sitting, we create tension and agitation. Over time, tension and agitation tire us out. Then we spend more muscle energy to prop ourselves up. As we tighten our core postural muscles to maintain an upright position, breathing becomes shallower. This decreases our energy further, inclining us to slump over. The cycle sustains itself.

When your spine is aligned naturally, it holds itself up. We need to supply some intention, but the energy expenditure is minimal. Two things have to happen in order for the spine to be in optimum alignment. First, your foundation (the parts of the body in contact with your cushion, bench, or chair) must be evenly and efficiently grounded. Next, your spinal curves must be intact. When these two conditions are met, while you may experience fatigue or agitation for reasons other than spinal misalignment, your body—and therefore your mind—has a much greater chance of finding equilibrium. Your sitting position then sustains, rather than depletes, energy.

The first step for creating a sustainable position is to determine what sitting position best allows for spinal congruence in your unique body. I will address five possibilities here: a zafu, a v-shaped cushion, a meditation bench, folded blankets, and a chair. You don't have to choose just one of these. If you are on a long meditation retreat, you may want to switch between a zafu and a chair, for example, if this fits within the guidelines of the retreat. In your home practice, you may find that a bench suits you on days when your energy is low, whereas a v-shaped cushion supports you better on days when you're feeling

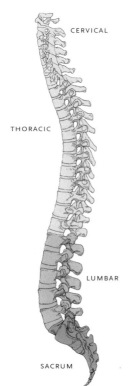

CERVICAL

THORACIC

LUMBAR

SACRUM

FIGURE 1.
VERTEBRAL COLUMN,
LATERAL VIEW

agitated. Staying open to shifts in your body-mind will help you determine what works best at a given time.

Most important, the position(s) you choose must support even grounding through your foundation and integrity of your natural spinal curves. The human spine, or vertebral column, develops with four natural curves. Two are convex; the other two are concave (Figure 1). These curves allow for shock absorption, and allow your spine to flex, extend, rotate, and side bend naturally as you move through space.

The two convex curves, in the sacrum and thorax, are stable, while the two concave curves, in the lumbar and cervical spine, are flexible. The concave curves give support to the structures immediately above them: the rib cage and head. When these curves are in integrity, the intervertebral discs create even space—front to back and side to side—between each vertebral body. When the vertebrae are evenly spaced, the discs stay healthy, not developing flat spots that can become brittle or bulging spots that can create pain by pushing out from between the vertebrae and impinging on nerves. When the vertebrae are in congruence, the discs create the cushion the spine needs to maintain its buoyancy and integrity.

In order to maintain these curves, we must focus our initial attention on the sacral angle. The sacral angle determines the ability of the rest of the spine to maintain its natural curves. The optimum angle for the sacrum is approximately 30 degrees, with the top of the sacrum angling forward.

There are a whole host of muscles and muscle groups that, when tight, can limit the sacrum's ability to find the magic angle. Tight hips, hamstrings, quadriceps, adductors, and abductors can all pull on the pelvis, causing it to tilt out of neutral, which usually brings the sacrum's angle to vertical, or can even cause the sacrum to tilt back. Postural habits such as constant tightening of the abdominal muscles can also affect the sacral angle and flatten the lumbar. All of these conditions not only make the spine unable to hold itself up easily, but over time they can also cause disc damage.

The even grounding of the sit bones is also essential. When we sit unevenly, with one sit bone more grounded than the other, the spine will misalign in whatever way it needs to for the body to stay upright.

Support is the key to bringing the spine to its optimum position. Even very flexible people don't do well sitting flat on the floor. So even if you have little restriction in the muscles that act on the pelvis and femur bones, using a bench, zafu, v-shaped cushion, chair, or blankets will allow you to sit more easily.

In our competitive Western culture, we often tend to see props as crutches. This is not at all the case—in yoga or in meditation. Using a cushion, bench, or chair in meditation simply allows you to create the most supportive position for sitting for long periods. You wouldn't want to run a marathon in flip-flops. Instead, you would wear shoes meticulously designed to help your body withstand the impact of constant pounding. The same applies to sitting. Struggling against the body is counterproductive in meditation. Even with the best support, you will likely experience challenges in your body when you sit. But if your spine is not aligned properly, struggle will be constant, and your nervous system will not be able to find equilibrium. Why not give yourself every possible opportunity to sit comfortably?

Selecting what you will sit on can take some experimentation. There are supports you can use for short meditation sessions that might not work for longer ones, and there are some that won't feel comfortable for you from the outset. You may try out something in a shop and find it perfectly comfortable, only to get it home and decide it's not the right choice for you. I sat on a meditation bench for my first several years of practice and then switched to sitting crosslegged. It took me a while to find the most comfortable position for long-term sitting, and I'm well aware that as time goes on I may shift yet again.

Here are guidelines for choosing a cushion or bench. When you decide to shop for a support, it might be helpful to bring along a friend who can assess whether your pelvis rests in the optimum angle on a cushion or bench. The illustrations in this section should help you understand what that looks like. Your most reliable feedback, of course, is your own body. Remember, feeling at ease and breathing freely is the most important cue. Explore all the options that work for your body, and be open to the possibility that over time your preferences may change.

Zafu

Zafus are round cushions, traditional to Japanese Zen meditation, with pleated or gathered sides. They are usually filled with either kapok or buckwheat hulls. Many zafus have openings so you can add or subtract filling to customize them to your body. One advantage of these cushions is that they are usually of a size and pliability that you can set them up to sit two different ways—cross-legged or kneeling.

If you choose to sit cross-legged (Figure 2), it's important that your knees be below your hip bones. If the knees are higher than the hip bones, with the thighbones angling upward, your pelvis will want to roll back. This flattens the lumbar curve. Also, the heads of the femur bones will press back into the sockets of the pelvis, which can cause discomfort and possibly wear and tear to the

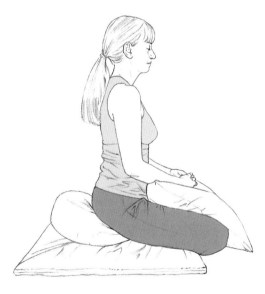

FIGURE 2.
SITTING CROSS-LEGGED ON A ZAFU,
WITH SHOULDER SUPPORT

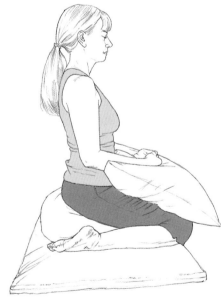

FIGURE 3.
KNEELING ON A ZAFU,
WITH SHOULDER SUPPORT

cartilage inside the sockets over time. For cross-legged sitting, it's best that the femur bones release down out of the sockets so that the hip joints can relax and the pelvis can tilt forward, bringing the sacrum into its optimum angle. If your hip flexibility allows you to sit with your knees below your hip bones and with your pelvis tilted forward, then a zafu might be a good choice for you.

You can also sit on the zafu in a kneeling position, with the cushion on edge between your thighs and shins (Figure 3). This position eliminates some of the outer and inner thigh restrictions that might prevent you from sitting cross-legged. Because the zafu offers two sitting options, it's the most versatile of all the choices.

On one long retreat, I discovered one disadvantage to sitting cross-legged on a zafu. The spot where my upper thighs met the edge of the zafu became extremely sensitive over time. The good news is that this only happened after about ten days of sitting six to eight hours a day, so it's quite possible this would never be a problem for you if you use the zafu for shorter daily sessions. The zafu has been around a very long time, so what happened to me may not happen to others, even over a long retreat. Still, I offer this issue as a possibility that might lead you to explore the next option, the v-shaped cushion.

V-Shaped Cushion

After the retreat where I experienced a lot of pain from sitting on the zafu, I decided to explore other possibilities. On my next thirty-day retreat, I tried a v-shaped cushion. For a person who prefers sitting cross-legged, the v-shaped cushion has all the advantages—height and variable filling (Figure 4). The pillow's shape allows the thighs to be supported evenly from the buttocks down to the knee, so there's no point where the thighs drop off an edge.

The v-shaped cushion is subject to all the conditions of cross-legged sitting on a zafu. Here again, the knees should be below the hip bones, and the spine should be able to maintain its natural curves. Indeed, the pillow's v shape won't really do you any good if your knees are high enough that the thighs don't rest on the "legs" of the cushion. The v-shaped cushion has been my favorite option since 1998.

Stacked Blankets

A stack of blankets can serve as a meditation cushion for yogis who can sit easily in a cross-legged position. Fold and stack two or more firm blankets so they are 4 to 6 inches high. Turn them so that one of the corners is facing forward. Then sit on the corner of the blanket with your thighs relaxing off the edges (Figure

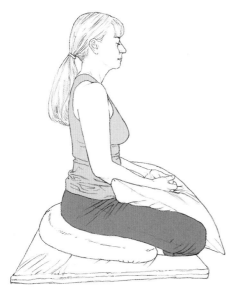

FIGURE 4.
SITTING CROSS-LEGGED ON A V-SHAPED
CUSHION, WITH SHOULDER SUPPORT

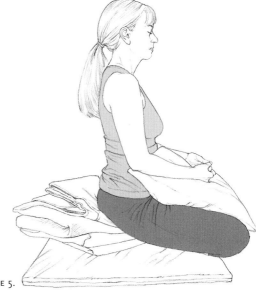

FIGURE 5.
SITTING CROSS-LEGGED ON STACKED
BLANKETS, WITH SHOULDER SUPPORT

5). I find this especially useful when I'm in a situation where I haven't brought my meditation cushion along—in a yoga class or when I'm out of town.

Meditation Bench

The meditation bench can be a great choice for anyone, regardless of flexibility or inflexibility (Figure 6). These low benches slant forward, so the pelvis can easily rest in a forward tilt. The bench is designed so you can fold your legs underneath, and most benches are high enough that people with tight quadriceps muscles (and therefore not-so-bendable knees) can sit comfortably. Still, some people with knee problems find the angle of the bend to be too much. Most people find it easy to ground their sit bones evenly when they sit on a bench.

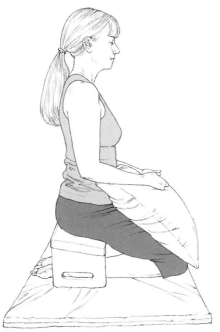

FIGURE 6. SITTING ON A MEDITATION BENCH, WITH SHOULDER SUPPORT

I sat on a bench for three years before switching to sitting cross-legged. Two things led me to switch. My sit bones are pretty close to the surface, and over time, no matter how much padding I put on my bench, my sit bones began to feel very tender. As with the zafu, this discomfort did not come with regular everyday sitting; it became apparent only on longer retreats.

My second reason for switching to cross-legged sitting was more energetic in nature. On a retreat in 1992, I began experiencing extreme agitation. While I was no stranger to agitation in meditation, this was different. I felt as if my body was in a monumental struggle against itself. Finally, after two days of extreme discomfort, I moved from my meditation bench to sitting cross-legged on blankets. Immediately, I felt at ease.

Here's why. At the time, I had just started my menstrual period. During menses, the *apana vayu*—one of the body's five natural energy flows recognized by the system of yoga—is predominant. *Apana* is a downward-moving energy that governs elimination. Sitting on a bench supports an upward-moving flow of energy. This can be very helpful for people who tend to get sleepy or sluggish in meditation. But for some women—not all—sitting on a bench during menses can create an uncomfortable energetic struggle. If you really enjoy sitting on a bench but it doesn't work for you during menstruation, you might want to switch to sitting some other way just during your period.

Zabuton

A zabuton is like a small futon, 3 to 4 inches thick, that provides extra padding under your knees or ankles. Place it under your zafu, v-shaped cushion, or meditation bench. Using a zabuton is optional, but I recommend it especially if you think you will be sitting for long periods. A bare floor, even with carpet, can feel harsh under your knees or ankle bones. A zabuton is a worthwhile luxury.

Chair

Ah, the chair. Sometimes a person's knees, hips, and back just need a break. While most chairs are not ergonomically designed for sitting with a neutral spine, with a little awareness and intention they can be just as supportive for meditation as any of the other options. Sitting in a chair is the best choice for people whose knees can't sustain being bent more than 90 degrees. It is also easier on many people's backs, as long as they take care to sit in a way that allows for spinal integrity. Like the meditation bench, a chair easily allows for an evenly grounded foundation.

As in sitting on a zafu or v-shaped cushion, the key to sitting in a chair with a neutral spine is having your knees below the hip bones (Figure 7). Begin by sitting on the front edge of the chair with your hips fully on the chair and thighs off the chair. Place your feet flat on the floor, directly below or a little behind your knees. The thighs should slant slightly downward. You may want to place one

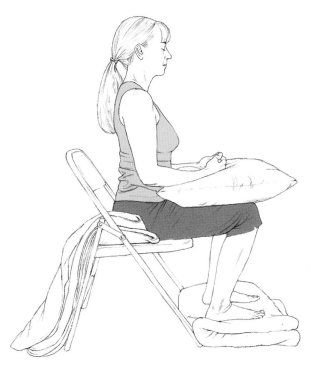

FIGURE 7. SITTING ON A CHAIR, WITH HIP, FOOT, AND SHOULDER SUPPORT

or more folded blankets under your hips to accomplish this. If you are short in stature, you may want to place a folded blanket under your feet to raise them so they can rest flat on the floor. Check your spinal position. If your sacrum is not slanting forward, you may want to use a foam wedge to create a pelvic tilt.

It may take you a while to find the best position for your body. Experiment with different chairs and different combinations of props. If you are on a retreat, the chair you use may be quite different from your chair at home. It's worth it to play with your position to find the most easeful way of sitting for your body.

Shoulder Support

One last helpful prop can ease some of the shoulder discomfort that often accompanies meditation. When the full weight of your arms hangs off your shoulders, the muscles on the tops of your shoulders can become very taut. Placing a cushion—a throw pillow works nicely—in your lap to support your forearms and hands will allow your shoulders to be softer and more mobile (Figures 2 through 7).

Make sure that your upper arms hang straight down from your shoulders rather than angling forward. When the arms angle forward, their weight can pull your entire torso forward. Again, play with what you use as support in order to find the most comfortable position.

Refining Your Position: The Active Yield

As long as we inhabit this earth, we are subject to the force of gravity. And it's a good thing. Without gravity we'd all be floating, untethered, out in space. Despite the everyday fact of gravity, we often seem to relate to this grounding force in unhealthy—and energy-sapping—ways.

According to Body-Mind Centering teacher Bonnie Bainbridge Cohen, we relate to gravity in three ways: collapsing, propping, and active yield. I invite you to try an easy exercise to help you identify these three patterns. You're likely to find one or all of them to be familiar.

Stand in a neutral position with your feet hip-width apart, and then allow your body to slump forward, as if you are really exhausted. Bend your knees slightly, and let all your weight sink down into your feet. Let your body go limp, as if you have no skeleton. Now feel your breathing. Notice where the breath moves easily within your trunk—and where it doesn't. This is collapsing into gravity (Figure 8). Psychologically, collapsing can feel self-negating, as if you are overwhelmed by your environment and your life.

Now come back to a neutral standing position. Begin to squeeze your muscles around your bones, and push against the floor with your feet, as if you are propping yourself up away from the earth. Tighten your abdomen and buttock muscles. Notice where and how the breath moves within your torso. This is called propping (Figure 9). Propping expresses a me-against-the-world attitude, a struggle against your environment. This can eventually lead to exhaustion.

Now come back again to neutral. Yield your body weight into your feet. You may

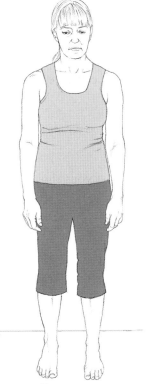

FIGURE 8. COLLAPSING: SLUMPING FORWARD

bend your knees slightly if it's helpful. Now actively press your feet into the floor even further, as if you are rooting them down into the ground. If your knees were bent, they will straighten now. You may feel a slight upward rebound in the upper body as you do this. This is called active yield (Figure 10).

Active yield is the same action you would do in order to jump—yield the weight, push the feet into the floor, and then lift off. But in active yield you

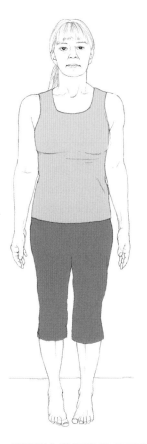

FIGURE 9. PROPPING: SQUEEZING AND TIGHTENING

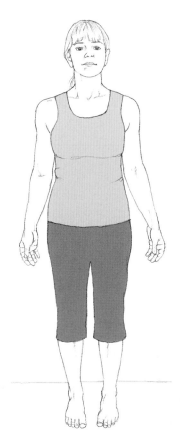

FIGURE 10. ACTIVE YIELD: STANDING

create the grounding action without actually jumping. You can try jumping a few times if this helps you to understand active yield a little better. Pay particular attention to the moment just before you leave the ground.

Using active yield in sitting practice has been tremendously helpful for me. In the previous section, I described a scenario where the body is careening back and forth between collapsing and propping. When you're shifting back and forth between the two extremes, your body becomes fatigued. In contrast, when you find active yield in your sitting position, there's a balance between upward and downward flowing energy in the body. In active yield, there's no futile struggle against gravity, and you can utilize your energy for your meditation rather than for trying to maintain your upright position.

Active yield in sitting happens most easily when you have aligned your pelvis and sit bones so that the spine can assume its natural curves. To find the center point of the sitting bones, where active yield is easy, sit in your meditation position, and roll the pelvis slowly and gently forward and backward, all the while pressing the sit bones into your cushion, bench, or chair (Figure 11). When you find the optimum position for your pelvis, you will feel an upward rebound in the torso as you ground your sit bones. You will also feel that you are centered within your torso, neither pushing forward into the

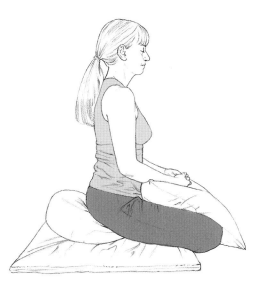

FIGURE 11. ACTIVE YIELD: SITTING

front body nor leaning back into the back body. This is the most supportive position for maintaining the quiet energy in the body that allows the mind to settle.

It is interesting to watch how the body tends to relate to gravity on a given day or at a given time. When we are tired, we tend to collapse. When we are stressed and agitated, or when we are struggling against discomfort in our meditation, we tend to prop. Setting the body in a balanced relationship to gravity—the active yield—creates the most supportive physical environment for the mind to relax, and it can alleviate sluggishness or agitation.

Asana for Meditation: Intentions for Practice

The results we reap from our practice depend on two factors: intention and action. When we practice poses that address specific meditation challenges, we are performing actions that will likely make our bodies less resistant to the rigors of sitting. Just as important is the intention we bring to our actions. Intention colors the results we receive as a consequence of performing an action. If you think of the poses as actions, your approach—the attitude you bring to practice—is your intention.

Just by shifting intention, we can practice the same pose but experience different results. If our intention is to accomplish a pose in a certain way, and we force ourselves right up to or over the edge of what our body can tolerate, we will achieve a particular result. If our intention is to bring mindful attention to each pose, to watch how it transforms naturally over time, we will experience a different result. If our intention is to quiet the nervous system to create a calm environment for our minds, we will reap yet a different result.

Three of the 196 verses in *The Yoga Sutras of Patanjali* are concerned with asana. The first one says (in Alistair Shearer's translation): "The physical posture should be steady and comfortable." Other translations use the words "firm and soft," "steady and easy," "alertness and relaxation." This means that whatever pose we're practicing embodies the seemingly disparate qualities of steadiness, commitment, and strength with ease, comfort, and relaxation.

To me, this implies a middle way, neither too strong nor too soft. Like the active yield, which is equal parts grounding and buoyancy, this intention helps create a balance between these two qualities of mind. The most reliable indicator for checking the quality of your intention in asana practice is your breath. A pose that is so forceful that it inhibits the movement of the breath through your torso will generate not energy but agitation. A pose that is collapsed, without tone, will create dullness rather than ease.

The mind and the breath are intimately connected. In order for the mind to settle, the breath must be steady and easy. The breath is the only autonomic function that we can easily control. Even though we breathe all day long without being conscious of it, we can take control of our breath if we want to create a specific effect on our physical or mental state. A slow, steady, full breath has a calming effect on the mind. Our asana practice can become a meditation in itself if we are conscious of and supportive of deep, complete breathing while we practice. When you practice meditation, it's helpful to spend a few minutes taking deep, slow breaths to help settle agitation in your mind.

In order to determine what full, relaxed breathing feels like in your body, lie on your back with your knees bent and the soles of your feet resting on the floor. You may want to place a small folded blanket or towel under your head and neck. Begin breathing deeply, allowing the belly to expand outward on your inhalation, and allowing it to rest back on the exhalation. Feel the expansion of the inhalation all the way down in the floor of your pelvis, between your sitting bones, allowing your pelvis to tilt forward naturally. The pelvis will likely want to tilt under slightly on the exhalation. Make sure you are not straining to breathe deeply. Stay in your comfort zone, but allow the breath to fill the torso completely on the in-breath. Check to see if you are attempting to hold the abdomen in as you inhale, and if you are, let the muscles relax. Exhale long and easy. (If you'd like to explore easeful breathing in more depth, read Donna Farhi's *The Breathing Book* [New York: Henry Holt, 1996].)

After you've imprinted what it feels like to breathe fully, apply this intention to your asana practice. A healthy asana will be a living, breathing entity rather than a static, frozen statue. Make sure there's enough play in your asana that your body can oscillate as you breathe. As you practice the asanas that follow, relax enough that your breath can be as full and easy as it was when you were lying down.

To that end, you may want to explore using props to help you. At the beginning of each asana description, I suggest helpful props. Try each pose, check your breathing, and if your breath is feeling restricted, use props to help you feel more ease in your pose. The illustrations that accompany the asana descriptions show how to use them. Of course, if you can feel steady and comfortable without props, you are free to practice the asanas sans support.

Part 2:

Yoga Poses for Sitting Meditation

▼　▼　▼　▼　▼　▼　▼　▼　▼　▼　▼　▼

Mountain Pose

TADASANA

▼ ▼ ▼ ▼ ▼ ▼ ▼ ESTABLISHES STABILITY WITH MOBILITY
ALIGNS NATURAL SPINAL CURVES • SUPPORTS DEEP BREATHING
IMPROVES BALANCE

PRACTICE WITH CARE: Practice on a firm, level surface.
If you have low blood pressure, do not stay in Mountain
Pose longer than 1 minute.

PROP: 1 nonskid mat

A mountain is a symbol of beauty and strength. Its beauty
lies in its towering granite peaks, solid brown earth,
fields of wildflowers, and cobalt-tinted snow. A mountain's strength comes from its ability to meet with grace
whatever comes its way. In a typical year, a mountain
weathers everything from the glaring, high-altitude sun
to gale-force winds and many feet of snow. In the spring,
the mountain becomes permeable, absorbing much of
the snowmelt and collecting the rest in crystalline lakes.
A mountain absorbs all that is visited upon it while maintaining its essential integrity.

In yoga, Mountain Pose (Figure 12) is the foundation

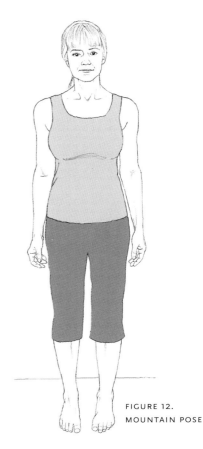

FIGURE 12.
MOUNTAIN POSE

for all the other asanas, especially the standing poses. When we align our structure in integrity, we become like a mountain—stable and solid, yet mobile and malleable. It may seem superfluous to spend time describing such a simple, basic pose—one that we do every day—but many of us have had natural, well-aligned posture taught out of us. Rather than nurturing our natural spinal curves, what many of us have been taught as correct posture actually flattens the curves. When we stand in Mountain Pose, as in sitting meditation, our spine rests in its natural curves and is able to move force easily, giving the posture both grounding and lightness. Mountain Pose is not only the basis for all the vertical postures in yoga practice, but it is also the best pose for standing meditation.

Begin by standing on your mat with your feet hip-width apart. Align the feet so they are parallel. Because the feet are wider at the toes than at the heel, the most accurate way to align the feet is to draw an imaginary line from a point between the second and third toes to the center of each ankle. Stand so those lines are parallel to each other.

Now become aware of the thighs. If you are like most people, your thighs are likely to be pushing forward. Draw the tops of the thighbones back slightly. If you press your fingers gently into the crease at the tops of the thighs (at the hip joint), the tendons and ligaments there should be slightly springy. For contrast, try pushing the thighs forward and tucking your tailbone. In this position, the tendons and ligaments of the hip joint will feel hard and tight. Draw the thighbones back until the tissue in the hip joints feels springy. It will probably feel as if your rear end is sticking out. It's not! It's just that we who grew up in Western culture have been taught to stand in a military position—with the tailbone tucked—which flattens out the sacral and lumbar curves. Allow your spine to be curvaceous!

Make sure you are not locking the knees. Locking often occurs because the thighs are pushing forward. Allowing the thighs and hip joints to release back will help bring the legs into a more vertical position. When the pelvis is in its proper neutral position, the knees are less likely to hyperextend.

As you ground (active yield) through the feet, allow your rib cage to lift gently, both front and back. Then allow your shoulder blades to slide slightly down the back toward your waist. As you inhale, your shoulder blades may move outward a bit. Allow that movement, as it mirrors the natural movement of the lungs on inhalation.

Now pay attention to your breathing. Mountain Pose, because it aligns the natural curves of the spine, supports deep breathing. For contrast, you can try tucking your tailbone and pulling your abdomen in. How does this change of posture affect your breathing? Then come back to Mountain Pose and take 5 to 10 deep, easy breaths.

Closing your eyes in Mountain Pose can help you understand and improve balance. Assume Mountain Pose and then close your eyes, letting the breath be easy and natural. Rest your attention on your feet, and feel what is happening in your feet as you stand, noticing all the little shifts taking place. Balancing is not about finding just the "right" position and then freezing there. You will likely find, as you pay attention, even in neutral standing, that your feet are making constant movements—side to side, forward and back, every which way—to keep you upright.

This is the nature of equilibrium or equanimity in our lives off the mat as well. Equanimity is the moment-to-moment mindful response to all the many and varied happenings in our lives. Standing mindfully in Mountain Pose can teach you about living an easeful life. Stay for 5 to 10 breaths, or longer if you are practicing standing meditation.

You can practice Mountain Pose almost anywhere: on your mat, in line at the grocery store or bank, for a few seconds when you get up from your desk at work, or when transitioning between sitting, walking, or lying down meditation—anytime, really. It is wonderful for centering yourself, especially at times when you feel scattered or anxious. In your asana practice, try moving into Mountain Pose between standing postures—kind of like coming home between poses. A mindful Mountain Pose in between other postures can teach you a lot about the effects of asana on your body-mind.

Tree Pose

VRKSASANA

▼ ▼ ▼ ▼ ▼ ▼ ▼ IMPROVES BALANCE
DEVELOPS CONCENTRATION

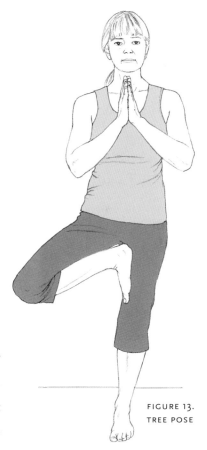

FIGURE 13.
TREE POSE

PRACTICE WITH CARE: Practice on a firm, level surface. Avoid it if you are experiencing dizziness. This pose is not recommended for women six months into pregnancy and beyond.

PROPS: 1 nonskid mat • a wall

Because they require concentration, balancing poses naturally collect the mind. Challenging your balance is a way of developing concentration. Balance poses are especially helpful when you come to your practice feeling scattered or agitated.

Begin by standing in Mountain Pose (Figure 12). Feel how the weight is distributed across your feet. Is there more weight on one foot, on the insides or outsides, or on the balls or heels? Also, feel how the feet shift and adjust to keep you balanced. The extent to which your feet need to move in order for you to balance will change from day to day, sometimes from minute to minute.

Settle your weight as evenly as possible over the feet, and practice active yield (as described on page 26). Shift your weight onto your right foot. Pick up the left ankle with your left hand, and place the foot on the right inner thigh. As you press the foot into the inner thigh, also press the inner thigh into the foot. If the left knee doesn't want to bend enough to allow your foot to press against your inner thigh, it's fine to place the left foot onto the right ankle or shin instead. Avoid pressing the left foot into the right knee.

When you feel balanced, place the palms together in Tree Pose (Figure 13), so your thumbs touch your breastbone. Stretch through the fingers and spread the palms. The contact of the palms should be steady and comfortable, so the hands are contacting each other evenly but not pressing hard. Check your breathing. Relax your body around the breath. Stay for 5 to 10 breaths. Come back to Mountain Pose, and notice how the two sides of the body feel. Repeat on the other side.

If balancing is a challenge for you, there are several options. First, you can place your left heel against your right ankle with your left big toe, second toe, and maybe third toe touching the floor. Or you can stand with your back at a wall, with your buttocks either close to or lightly touching the wall.

One more hint for balancing poses: The mind's attention is often drawn to the parts of the body that are changing position rather than the parts that are stationary. When this happens in a balancing pose, you lose mental contact with the standing leg. This can interfere with your ability to stay upright. Set an intention to give the lion's share of your attention to the leg you are standing on. As you move into and out of the pose, stay present with the sensations in the standing foot and leg.

Eagle Pose

GARUDASANA

▼ ▼ ▼ ▼ ▼ ▼ ▼ DEVELOPS CONCENTRATION
LENGTHENS HIP ROTATORS • EXPANDS UPPER BACK

PRACTICE WITH CARE: Practice on a firm, level surface. If you have knee problems, do not attempt to curl your ankle around the calf of your standing leg. Use caution if you have shoulder or upper back injuries. Not recommended in pregnancy beyond six months.

PROPS: 1 nonskid mat • a wall • 1 strap

Begin in Mountain Pose (Figure 12). As with all standing asanas, Eagle Pose (Figure 14) begins with becoming aware of how your feet contact the floor. Take a moment to check. Do you feel more weight on one foot, or on the balls or heels, or on the insides or outsides? Shift your weight so you feel as even as possible.

Bend your knees about 45 degrees, letting your weight settle into your feet. Shift your weight onto

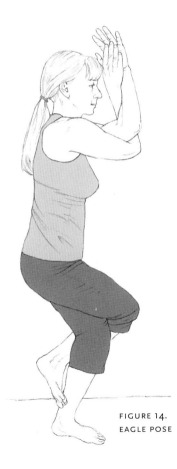

FIGURE 14.
EAGLE POSE

your right foot, and then cross your left thigh over the right thigh. If you can, hook the left ankle behind the right calf. Otherwise, flex the left foot and let it dangle. When you feel steady in your balance, cross the right upper arm over the left, and then place the fingers of the left hand into the palm of your right hand. If your fingers can't reach the right palm, use a strap to connect your hands. Direct your breath into your back body. Take 5 to 10 breaths. Return to Mountain Pose. Take a few breaths to check in with your feet, legs, shoulders, and back body. Do your legs feel different from each other? What sensations do you experience in the area between the shoulder blades? Repeat on the other side.

A general rule to remember here is if the right leg is crossing over the left leg, the left upper arm will cross over the right, and vice versa.

STANDING SIDE BEND

▼ ▼ ▼ ▼ ▼ ▼ RELIEVES BODILY TENSION

PRACTICE WITH CARE: Practice on a firm, level surface. Be especially careful if you have shoulder or neck injuries.

PROPS: 1 nonskid mat • 1 strap

There's something especially satisfying about side bending. Standing Side Bend (Figure 15) is not a traditional yoga asana, but it ought to be. Many of us do this movement intuitively when we want to unwind tension. It's a helpful pose to do before and after sitting meditation, or anytime during the day—first thing in the morning, or on breaks from your computer desk.

Stand on your mat in Mountain Pose (Figure 12). Hold a strap with both hands, shoulder-width apart or wider. Adjust the distance between your hands to see what feels best for you on a given day. I like to loop the strap around my hands so I don't have to grip tightly. Raise your arms above your head. Ground your right foot by extending the leg downward. Exhale, bending the body over to the

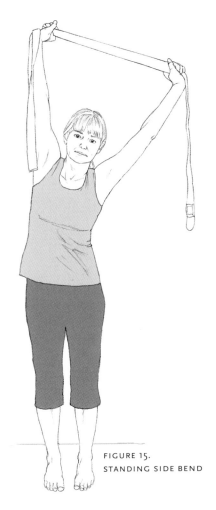

FIGURE 15.
STANDING SIDE BEND

left, taking care not to hunch your right shoulder up toward your right ear. Breathe deeply into the right side of the body, especially the waist and rib cage. You can either stay in this position or play with rotating the trunk forward or back slowly and mindfully. Breathe deeply and continuously. After 5 to 10 breaths, come back to Mountain Pose. Repeat on the other side.

Wall Dog Pose

ADHO MUKHA SVANASANA

▼ ▼ ▼ ▼ ▼ ▼ ▼ REVITALIZES TIRED ARMS • RELIEVES SORE
SHOULDERS • STRETCHES HAMSTRINGS • LENGTHENS TORSO
ENCOURAGES DEEP BREATHING

PRACTICE WITH CARE: Practice slowly and gently if you have lower back, hamstring, or shoulder injuries. If you are nursing any of these injuries, walk your hands up the wall so they are higher than hip level and your trunk is slanted.

PROPS: 1 nonskid mat • a wall

Like Standing Side Bend (Figure 15), this is a perfect 1-minute stretch break at work, in addition to providing an excellent all-over stretch to complement sitting practice. A variation of Downward-Facing Dog Pose, Wall Dog Pose (Figure 16) is one

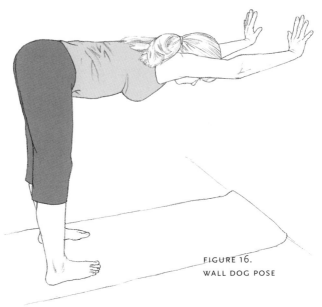

FIGURE 16.
WALL DOG POSE

of my favorite poses to do first thing in the morning. I like to practice it with my hands on my countertop while my tea water is heating.

Stand in Mountain Pose (Figure 12), a few feet from the wall. On an exhalation, bend forward and place your palms flat against the wall. Walk your feet forward or back, so the legs become vertical. Reach one hand back, and place your fingers on your lumbar spine. If you feel the knobby spinous processes poking out in your lower back, walk your hands up the wall a few inches. When the spinous processes poke out, it's a signal that your lumbar spine is in a convex, rather than concave, curve. Continue walking your hands up the wall until you feel an indentation, kind of like a gutter, in the lumbar area. It can be helpful to enlist a friend to help you determine how high your hands need to be in order for your spine to be in neutral position. (See Figure 1 for an illustration of the spinal curves.)

Press your hands into the wall, and ground through your feet. If your feet are too close to the wall, you will "float" away from the wall when you press through your hands. If your feet are too far away, you will feel as if you are leaning into the wall. Find a distance from the wall that allows you to feel your hips stretching back as you push forward into the wall.

Particularly if your back is flexible, you may find your rib cage hanging down toward the floor. (If back bending is easy for you, this is something you should be aware of.) Take care not to let the rib cage collapse down toward the floor. Instead, lengthen the torso, drawing the internal organs back toward the spine, so the stretch is continuous throughout your trunk—front, back, and through your core.

Take 5 to 10 deep breaths as you actively yield through the hands and feet.

To come out of Wall Dog Pose, bend your elbows and walk your feet forward to lift up to Mountain Pose. Repeat if you like.

If you don't have a free wall available, you can do this with your palms flat on a horizontal surface such as a desk, the back of a chair, or a countertop. In this position, you won't have the benefit of pushing into the wall, but you can root your feet and extend your hips back for a lovely shoulder release.

Wide-Leg Standing Forward Bend Pose
PRASARITA PADOTTANASANA

▼ ▼ ▼ ▼ ▼ ▼ ▼ RELAXES THE UPPER BODY
STRETCHES AND ENERGIZES THE LEGS

PRACTICE WITH CARE: If you have concerns about your head being below your heart because of untreated high blood pressure, glaucoma, or a detached retina, place a block under your hands so your back stays horizontal. You should also use a block in this way if you have diagnosed disc problems.

PROPS: 1 nonskid mat • 1 block

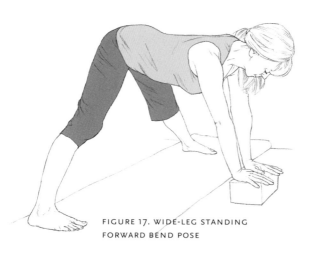

FIGURE 17. WIDE-LEG STANDING FORWARD BEND POSE

Most people don't think of standing poses as cooling or relaxing, but Wide-Leg Standing Forward Bend Pose (Figure 17) has both of these qualities, and more. It can help your legs feel more relaxed in sitting meditation, and after sitting this pose can help "wake up" your legs. Like most standing poses, the legs are strong and active here, which allows the upper body to relax.

Begin on your mat in Mountain Pose (Figure 12). Bend your knees and jump your feet out wide so the distance between them approximates the length of your legs (3 feet or more). If you prefer not to jump, you may step your feet out wide to a leg's length apart. Turn your feet so your big toes point slightly toward each other, and straighten your knees. With your elbows bent, place your hands on your outer hips, at the place where the legs join the trunk.

Keeping the spine long, exhale and bend the trunk forward from the pelvis, stretching out through the legs and grounding the feet. Make sure that as you bend forward, your pelvis tips forward along with your spine. When you begin to feel your hamstrings stretching, allow your hands to rest on the floor. If they do not reach the floor, place a block under your hands. Now allow your spine to hang forward as you breathe slowly and gently into your back. Relax your neck, allowing your head to hang. Let your facial muscles relax so they slide up toward your forehead, kind of like a shar-pei dog. Take 5 to 10 deep breaths here.

To come out of the forward bend, place the inner edges of your hands, the webs between the thumbs and index fingers, into the creases where your thighs meet your pelvis. Press back into the creases, and inhale as you lift up to standing, keeping your spine, neck, and head straight, relaxed, and easy. If you feel dizzy when you come up to standing, bend forward again, this time bending your knees and resting your hands on your knees for a few deep breaths. Then lift back up to standing.

You can ask a friend to help you find a neutral position for your spine. It is okay for your spine to round in this pose, as long as the pelvis is tilting forward and your hands are resting on the floor or on a block. But if your pelvis is tilting back and you are bending from your waist, you may put unhealthy pressure on the front of some of your lumbar discs.

Extended Triangle Pose
UTTHITA TRIKONASANA

▼ ▼ ▼ ▼ ▼ ▼ ▼ INVIGORATES THE LEGS • OPENS THE HIP JOINT
RELAXES THE BACK • LENGTHENS THE ARMS • EXPANDS THE CHEST

PRACTICE WITH CARE: This pose is not recommended at times when your balance is shaky: during your menstrual period, during or after an illness, or in the last six weeks of pregnancy. You can practice with your back against a wall for extra support.

PROPS: 1 nonskid mat • 1 block

Extended Triangle Pose (Figure 18) expresses strength and expansion. It's a staple of asana practice and, from my unscientific surveys of students over the years, is the hands-down favorite of all the standing poses, because it feels really good.

Stand in Mountain Pose (Figure 12). Bend your knees, and jump your feet out wide so the distance between them approximates the length of your legs (3 feet or more). If you prefer, you may step your feet out wide to a leg's length apart. Turn your left foot in slightly, so it's at about a 30-degree angle turning toward your right foot. Turn your entire right leg out, so your foot points straight out and the centers of your ankle, knee, and thigh are aligned with each other. Now

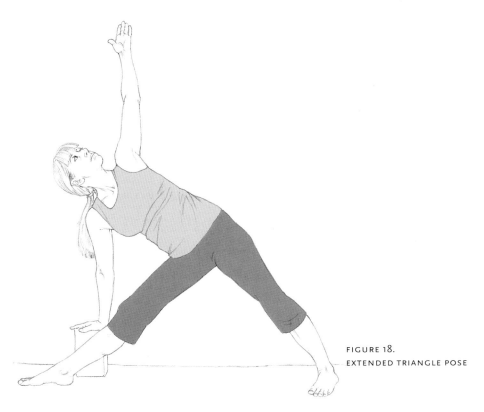

FIGURE 18.
EXTENDED TRIANGLE POSE

ground your left foot, and begin rolling your left hip slightly inward until you feel a clear line of force through your left leg. When your hips are at the optimum angle, your back foot will feel solidly rooted into the floor.

Use active yield to create a balance between grounding and lightness: On an exhalation, with your hands on your hips, bend your knees slightly, and yield your weight into your feet. Then, in order to straighten the legs, press the feet into the floor, as if you're sending down roots.

On an inhalation, raise your arms in front of you, shoulder-width apart, up to shoulder level, and then extend them out to the sides, straight out from your shoulders. Allow your shoulder blades to slide down your back toward the pelvis, so that your neck stays long.

With both feet firmly and evenly grounded, inhale, and on your exhalation extend your right arm and torso out to the right side, lengthening the waist and rib cage as you go. Let the pelvis move back slightly to the left, as you lengthen out through the trunk. Place your right hand on your ankle, shin, or a block. Notice if you tend to collapse into the right hand; that can bring a sluggish energy to your upper body. Instead, practice active yield through your right hand by pressing it into the block or floor. It is important that your torso be in a neutral position, so its two sides are equally long, extending straight out and not bowing upward. If your hamstrings are especially resistant, and a block is not high enough to allow your torso to be neutral and easy, you can place your hand on the seat of a chair.

Extend the left arm up toward the ceiling, keeping it vertical. While it might be tempting to throw the arm back past vertical, keep it aligned with your chest, with the palm facing forward. Let your head face forward and relax your eyes and jaw. Take several deep breaths. (If you like to turn your head upward in this pose, do so during your last breath or two, taking care not to strain your neck.) In Extended Triangle Pose, as in all the asanas, allow your body to oscillate as you breathe, so your posture reflects the internal movements of your breath.

To come back up, on an exhalation ground your back foot, and inhale to lift your torso back up to upright. Turn your feet to parallel and take a few breaths, feeling the effects of the pose. Turn your feet to the other side, again being mindful of your foot and leg alignment, and repeat. Remember to bend from the hips in Extended Triangle Pose. Your pelvis should move with the spine when you extend to each side.

Warrior I Pose

VIRABHADRASANA I

▼ ▼ ▼ ▼ ▼ ▼ ▼ STRENGTHENS QUADRICEPS
STRETCHES CALF MUSCLES • PROMOTES A FLEXIBLE SPINE
GENERATES ENERGY AND HEAT

PRACTICE WITH CARE: This pose can be overly heating during your menstrual period, so it is best not to practice it during this time. It is also not recommended at times when your balance is shaky or during or after an illness. Because it is a back bend, do not practice it in the later months of pregnancy, as it may cause abdominal pressure.

PROPS: 2 nonskid mats (1 optional)

Stand in Mountain Pose (Figure 12) on one end of your mat. Step your left leg straight back about 4 feet. Turn your left foot out, but only slightly. Square your chest toward the wall in front of you. Ground the left heel, shifting your weight back toward the left leg. On an inhalation, raise your arms up in front of you, and then lift them toward the ceiling. Soften your throat so it feels spacious, and look straight ahead so the back of your neck feels long. On an exhalation, bend the right knee to about 90 degrees and come into Warrior 1 Pose (Figure 19). If your knee bends so that it extends beyond the heel, widen your stance so the knee is directly over your heel.

The right knee may not bend that deeply, but don't worry. Bend it to where it feels strong and comfortable. Also, the left heel may want to come off the floor. If this is the case, place a second rolled-up, nonskid mat under your heel; if you don't have one, let the heel come up. Do not turn the heel out in order to ground it. This could cause an unhealthy torque in your left knee. Whether your heel is in contact with something or not, extend strongly back through the left leg.

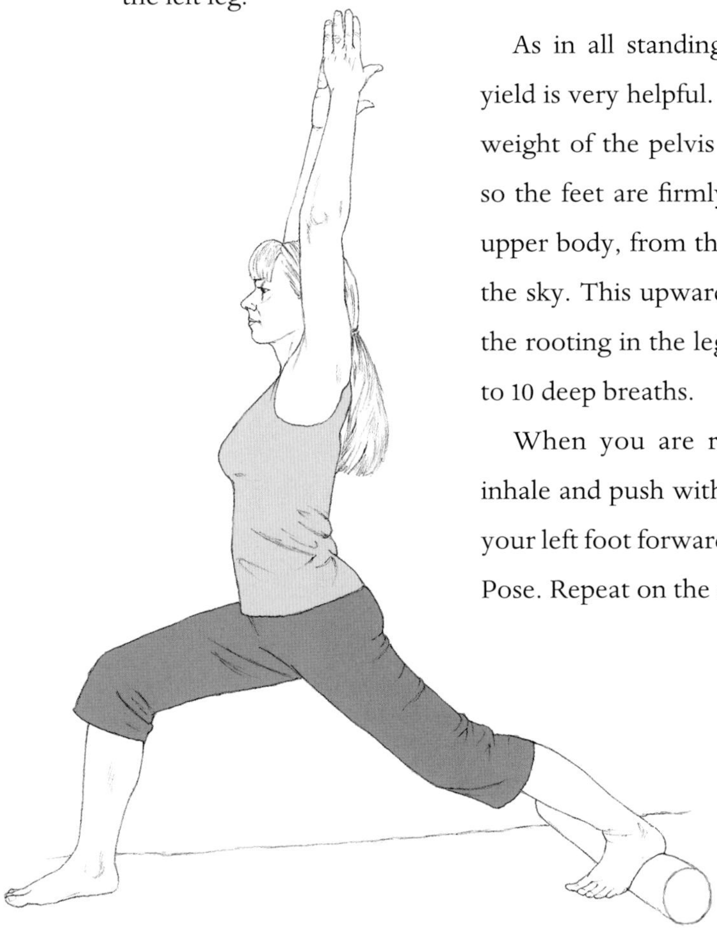

As in all standing poses, practicing active yield is very helpful. In Warrior I Pose, let the weight of the pelvis feed down into the legs, so the feet are firmly grounded. Then let the upper body, from the waist up, fly up toward the sky. This upward movement comes from the rooting in the legs. Stay in Warrior I for 5 to 10 deep breaths.

When you are ready to leave the pose, inhale and push with your feet to lift up. Step your left foot forward, and return to Mountain Pose. Repeat on the other side.

FIGURE 19. WARRIOR I POSE

Extended Side-Angle Pose

UTTHITA PARSVAKONASANA

▼ ▼ ▼ ▼ ▼ ▼ ▼ ENERGIZES THE BODY
STRENGTHENS THE LEGS • IMPROVES BALANCE

PRACTICE WITH CARE: This pose is contraindicated in the later stages of pregnancy, six months and beyond, and during your menstrual period. If you choose to practice Extended Side-Angle Pose when you are shaky or recovering from an illness, practice with your back against a wall.

PROPS: 1 nonskid mat • 1 block • a wall

Extended Side-Angle Pose (Figure 20) is not only lovely to look at, but it is also especially invigorating for the entire body after sitting in meditation or at a desk. Begin standing on your mat in Mountain Pose (Figure 12). If you are using a wall for stability, stand with your heels about 6 inches from the wall. Step or jump your feet out about 4 feet. As in Extended Triangle Pose (Figure 18),

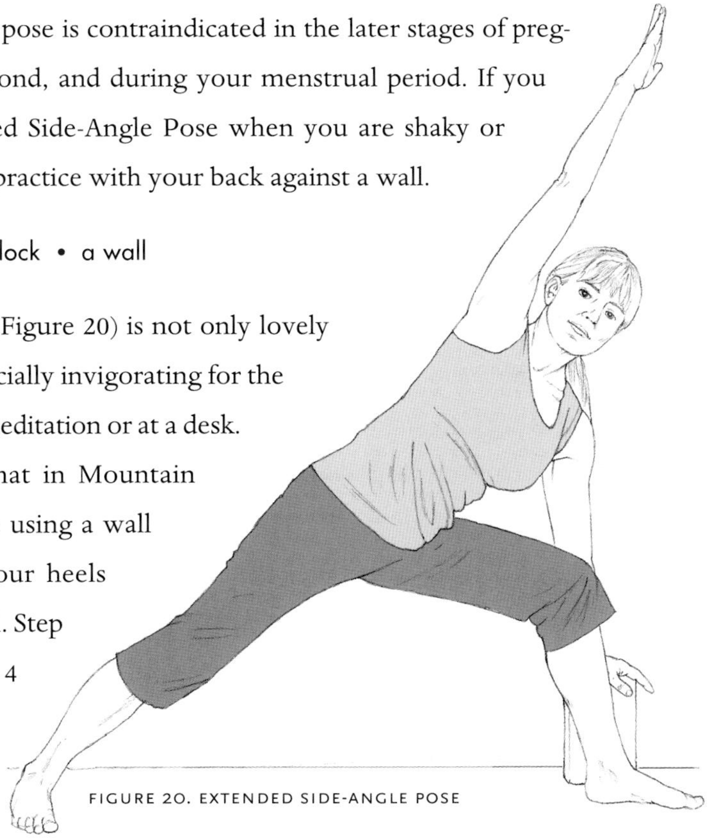

FIGURE 20. EXTENDED SIDE-ANGLE POSE

turn your left leg and foot out, so the centers of the ankle, knee, and thigh are all pointing straight out. Turn your right foot in toward the right foot about 30 degrees. At the same time, as in Extended Triangle Pose, allow your right hip to rotate inward until you feel a strong grounding through your right foot. Practice active yield by bending both knees slightly and letting your weight sink into your feet. Then press the feet into the floor to straighten the knees.

Inhale and sweep the arms forward, up to shoulder level, and then out to the sides. On an exhale, ground through your right foot and bend your left knee to a right angle, making sure that your knee does not extend past your heel. If it does, widen your stance so the knee is directly over your heel. Extend your left arm and torso out over the left leg, still grounding strongly through your right foot. Place your elbow on your left thigh, pressing the elbow into the thigh to help you rotate your trunk up to look forward. Extend your right arm, palm down, alongside your head, so there is a continuous line of extension along the entire right side of the body, from the foot to the fingertips.

If you can place your left hand on a block or on the floor (on the outside of your left foot) without inhibiting your breath or losing the continuous line on the right side of the body, feel free to experiment with it. Practice active yield through your left hand by extending it down into the block or floor. The tendency is to lean into the hand, which de-energizes the pose, so make sure you are practicing active yield to keep the pose vital.

Stay in Extended Side-Angle Pose for 5 to 10 deep breaths. When you are ready to return to standing, press both feet into the floor, allowing the upper body to spring back to upright. If you are using a block, bring it along so you can use it for your second side. Turn your feet so they are parallel to each other, and rest in the middle for a few breaths. Repeat on your second side.

Gate Latch Pose

PARIGHASANA

▼ ▼ ▼ ▼ ▼ ▼ ▼ STRETCHES THE SIDE BODY, INCLUDING THE LOW, MIDDLE, AND UPPER TORSO • OPENS THE SHOULDER JOINTS

PRACTICE WITH CARE: This pose is contraindicated in the later stages of pregnancy, six months and beyond, because of the strong stretch to each side of the abdomen.

PROPS: 1 nonskid mat • 1 block • 1 blanket

Gate Latch Pose (Figure 21) is another exquisite side stretch. Unlike Extended Triangle Pose (Figure 18) and Extended Side-Angle Pose (Figure 20), where the pelvis moves with the spine, here the pelvis roots into the legs, creating a true lateral extension.

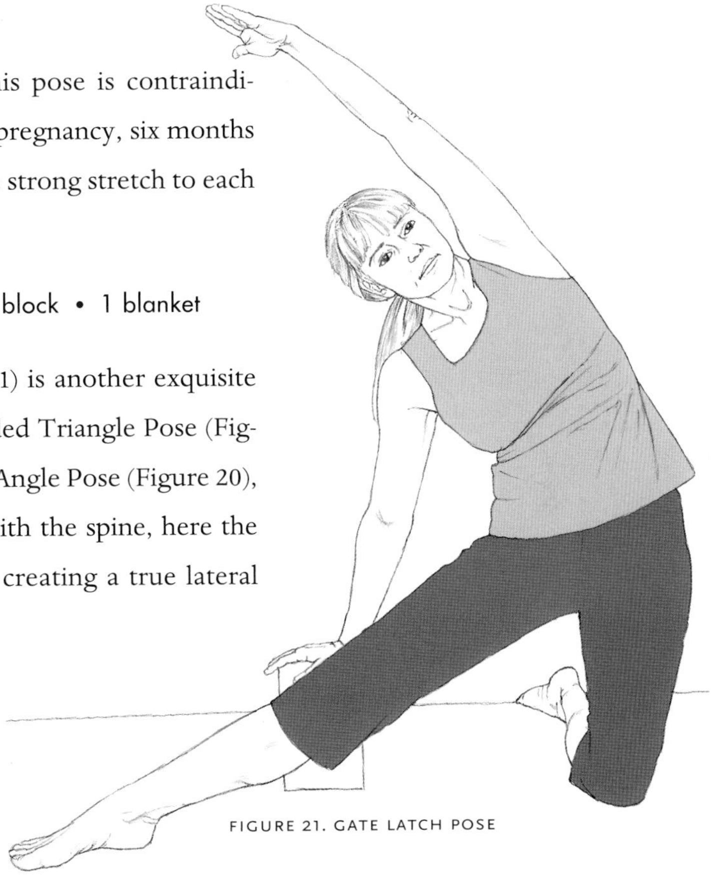

FIGURE 21. GATE LATCH POSE

Kneel on your mat with your thighs hip-width apart so your shins and feet point straight back. (For comfort, you can place a blanket, folded to 1 inch thick, lengthwise on your mat. Kneel on the blanket so your knees, shins, and feet are supported.) Extend your right leg out to the right side, allowing it to angle slightly inward. Rotate the leg so the centers of the ankle, knee, and thigh are all facing straight upward. Press out through the ball of your right foot so the ball of the foot is on, or moving toward, the floor.

Inhale and raise the left arm forward and up toward the ceiling alongside your head. Exhale and rotate your rib cage slightly toward the left. Inhale, and on the exhalation, ground through your left shin as you extend your trunk out over the right leg. Place your right hand on a block, and practice active yield through the right hand, as in Extended Triangle Pose and Extended Side-Angle Pose. Direct the weight of the pelvis down into the left knee and shin as you extend the entire left side of the torso and lengthen out through the fingertips. Take 5 to 10 deep, full breaths, allowing the body to oscillate along with your inhalations and exhalations. On an inhalation, ground through the left knee and shin to come up. Repeat on the second side.

Basic Lunge Pose

ARDHA MANDALASANA

▼ ▼ ▼ ▼ ▼ ▼ ▼ REVITALIZES THE LEGS
STRETCHES THE QUADRICEPS • CREATES FLEXIBILITY IN THE SPINE

PRACTICE WITH CARE: If you have sacroiliac issues or are pregnant, stay well inside your comfort zone when practicing lunges. Avoid letting your pelvis sink toward the floor.

PROPS: 1 nonskid mat • 1 blanket • 2 blocks

To begin, stand in Mountain Pose (Figure 12) at one end of your mat. Place the webs between your thumbs and index fingers into the hip joints, where the thighs meet the pelvis. Pressing back into the hip joints, exhale and bend from the pelvis, allowing the lumbar spine to bend forward so your head and shoulders lengthen downward toward the floor. Bend your knees to whatever degree is necessary for your hands to touch the floor. Lengthen the back of your neck so the top of your head releases toward the floor. Then press the left foot and both hands into the floor, and step the right leg back, resting your right knee on the floor and keeping the toes turned under. Make sure your stance is wide enough that your left knee is directly over your heel (as in Warrior I Pose, Figure 19). (Place a folded blanket under your knee if your kneecap feels uncomfortable on your mat.) Relax your torso onto the left thigh in Basic Lunge Pose (Figure 22). Take 5 to 10 deep breaths, continuing to relax your torso onto your thigh. To come out, press through the ball and toes of the right foot, and push off to step forward. Relax here for a few breaths before coming up and then moving to your second side.

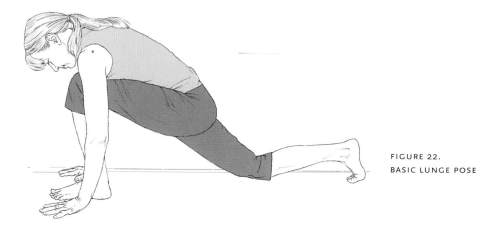

FIGURE 22.
BASIC LUNGE POSE

You can vary Basic Lunge Pose in lots of ways. I've given you three here. For each, begin and end as for Basic Lunge Pose. Feel free to have fun with them!

Variation 1. Press the right knee into the floor, as you lengthen the spine and lift your torso off the left thigh, so you are facing forward and looking straight ahead (Figure 23). You can place your hands on blocks to create greater freedom to lift the spine.

Variation 2. Turn the toes of your right foot under, and straighten your right leg, lifting the knee off the floor (Figure 24). Press your hands into the floor (or blocks), and stretch through your right heel.

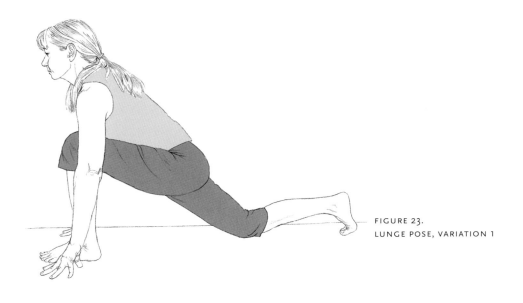

FIGURE 23.
LUNGE POSE, VARIATION 1

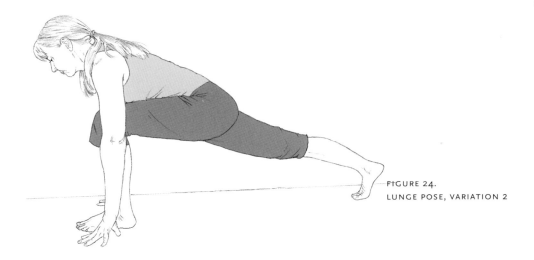

FIGURE 24.
LUNGE POSE, VARIATION 2

Variation 3. Thanks to Donna Farhi for this wonderful variation. Turn your left foot out 90 degrees, and scoot it back a bit, so it is even with your hip-bones. Rotate your torso to face the left knee, and press your left hand into the floor, using active yield. Place your right hand on your right hip and continue

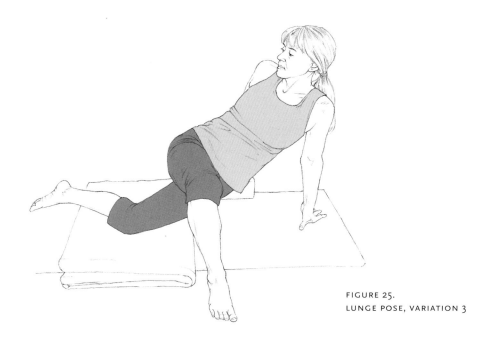

FIGURE 25.
LUNGE POSE, VARIATION 3

rotating, breathing deeply (Figure 25). If your arms are long, you may be able to place your right hand behind you on the floor or on a block. If this is the case, press your hand into the block or floor to help you rotate a bit more. Take 5 to 10 breaths before unwinding back to the center, turning your left foot to face forward again.

One-Leg King Pigeon Pose
EKA PADA RAJA KAPOTASANA

▼ ▼ ▼ ▼ ▼ ▼ ▼ STRETCHES THE ABDUCTORS
STRETCHES THE HIP ROTATORS

PRACTICE WITH CARE: If you have knee problems or feel discomfort in your bent knee in the pose, sit on a block or folded blanket and open the bend of your front knee so it is moving toward 90 degrees. If this does not alleviate discomfort, then skip this pose for now.

PROPS: 1 nonskid mat • 1 to 3 blankets • 1 block

One-Leg King Pigeon Pose (Figure 26) is especially helpful in stretching the muscles that need to elongate in order for you to sit comfortably in a cross-

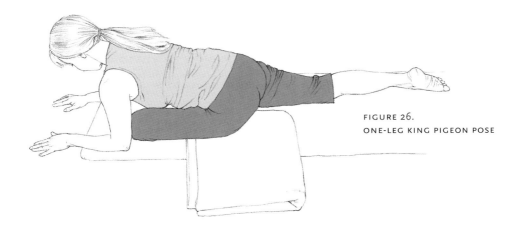

FIGURE 26.
ONE-LEG KING PIGEON POSE

legged position. It's a favorite among my yoga students for its ability to counteract the tightening effect of sitting in chairs, bicycling, and running.

Begin on your hands and knees on your mat. You can spread a blanket over your mat for extra cushioning. Slide your left knee forward, so it is next to your left thumb, and then rotate the leg slightly, so the left foot is under your right thigh or hip. Slide your right leg back, so it is almost straight. Lower your hips to wherever they are willing—the hips will likely be anywhere from 1 inch to 5 or 6 inches from the floor—so your pelvic bones stay parallel to the floor.

If your hips are pretty flexible, your left buttock may reach the floor easily without compromising your alignment. But if your hips are less flexible, take advantage of your props, using one or more folded blankets to support your hip, so your body does not lean over to the left. If you feel that the weight in the back leg is on the inner side of the leg, you are probably leaning a bit to the left. In this case, place a folded blanket or a block under your left hip.

With your arms straight, press your hands into the floor (active yield), and take 5 or more breaths. Then, if you like, you can relax your torso over the right knee, resting your elbows and forearms on the floor. Take 5 or more breaths here. After you have finished the first side, return to all fours and check in with your hips, noting any differences between your two sides. Then practice the pose with your right leg forward and left leg back. The hips are one area of the body where your sides could be quite different, so adjust your props accordingly, using more or less height under your pelvis, as necessary.

Cross-Leg Revolved Pose

PARIVRTTA SUKHASANA

▼ ▼ ▼ ▼ ▼ ▼ ▼ ROTATES THE SPINE • EXPANDS THE CHEST
RELIEVES GENERAL BACK DISCOMFORT

PRACTICE WITH CARE: If you have knee problems, try placing a block or folded blanket under the injured knee. If you try this and your knee still does not feel comfortable, you may practice this twist sitting sideways in a chair. Twists are not recommended in the first trimester of pregnancy. In the second and third trimesters, stay well inside your edge (the farthest degree of your twist). For example, revolve about 10 percent less than you are able.

PROPS: 1 nonskid mat • 1 or more blankets, or a zafu or v-shaped meditation cushion

In addition to including Cross-Leg Revolved Pose (Figure 27) in an asana practice sequence, you can also practice it while sitting cross-legged on a

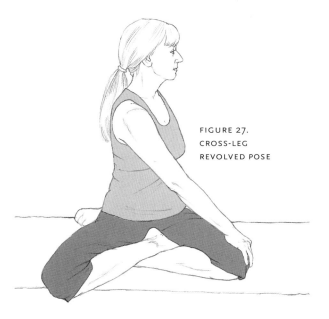

FIGURE 27.
CROSS-LEG
REVOLVED POSE

zafu or v-shaped cushion. Try practicing this pose just before you begin your sitting practice, at the end of your sitting session, or both. If your knees are higher than your hipbones in cross-legged position, you can practice this twist while sitting on a chair or meditation bench.

Sit cross-legged on your mat on one or more folded blankets (or a zafu or v-shaped cushion). Fold them so they are 4 to 6 inches thick, stack them, and turn them so you are sitting on one corner of the stack. Practice active yield by rooting your hips down into your blankets. Slide your right hip forward 1 or 2 inches as you turn your torso toward your left leg. Place your right hand on the outside of your left knee. At the same time, extend the right knee out to the right.

Make sure you are able to breathe easily here. If the breath feels restricted, turn slightly back toward the center, so you can feel the natural oscillation of the body as you inhale and exhale. (For most people, the body will move slightly out of the twist on the inhalation and move back into it on the exhalation.) Check in with your right arm. Are you pulling on your left leg to the point that you feel as if you are "doing the pose" to yourself? If so, relax the arm, and let it instead be a support to the natural rotational movement of your torso. Take 5 or more deep breaths. Turn back to the center, and take a few breaths in a neutral position before repeating the pose on the other side. Then come back to the center, cross your legs the opposite way, and repeat the twist on each side.

Chair Revolved Pose. If you prefer to sit on a chair instead of in a cross-legged position, place the chair near the edge of your mat and sit sideways on it. Instead of putting your hand on the knee you are turning toward, place both hands on the back of the chair to help you turn (Figure 28). Do not try to keep

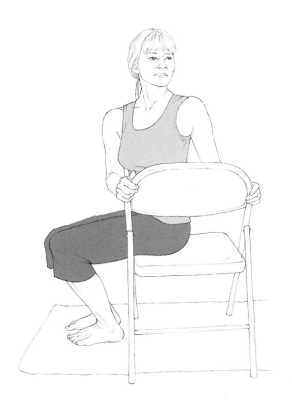

FIGURE 28. CHAIR REVOLVED POSE

the knees aligned with each other, as this can put unhealthy demands on your sacroiliac joint. Let the outside knee and hip slide forward, so the outer knee is a few inches in front of the inside knee. Take 5 or more deep breaths. When you are ready to practice your second side, turn 180 degrees on your chair, so your other side is next to the chair back.

Reclining Leg Stretch Pose
SUPTA PADANGUSTHASANA

▼ ▼ ▼ ▼ ▼ ▼ ▼ STRETCHES THE HAMSTRINGS • STRETCHES THE
INNER THIGHS

PRACTICE WITH CARE: If your head tilts back so your chin is higher than your forehead when you lie on your back, place a pillow or folded blanket under your head to make it level. Avoid practicing in the second and third trimesters of pregnancy.

PROPS: 1 nonskid mat • a wall • 1 blanket • 1 strap

Reclining Leg Stretch Pose (Figure 29) targets the hamstrings and inner thighs without causing stress in the spine. For this reason, I often recommend this pose to people with disc problems who want to stretch their hamstrings safely. We'll practice the basic pose and a variation.

Spread your mat on the floor so the short end touches the wall. For extra comfort, you can place a blanket over the length of the mat. Lie on your back on the mat with your legs extended and your feet against the wall. With the rim of your heels on the floor, press both feet into the wall. Now press your left foot into the wall as you bend your right knee and draw it toward you. Use both hands to hold on to the right leg, either around the shin or behind the knee.

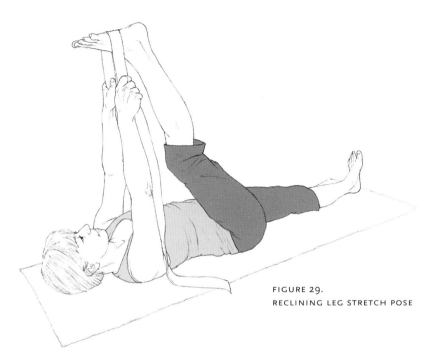

FIGURE 29.
RECLINING LEG STRETCH POSE

Notice if your left leg lifts off the floor or if you lose the grounding of your left foot against the wall when you draw your right leg in. If so, reground the back of the left leg against the floor by lengthening the back of your leg, and press your foot into the wall. In this pose, the grounding of the stabilizing leg is just as important as the stretching of the other leg. Give your grounding leg as much of your intention as you give your stretching leg.

Loop a strap around your right foot, and extend your right leg so the knee is straight and you are feeling a stretch in your hamstrings. Hold your strap with both hands, arms extended. Give yourself enough slack in the strap so your knee can be straight. Don't worry about the angle of the right leg to the body. Let it be at whatever angle gives you a full stretch with the leg straight. Relax your abdomen and breathe deeply, allowing the body to oscillate with the breath. If the right leg wants to move away from you on the inhalation, allow it to do so; if it wants to draw back in on the exhalation, allow this also.

It's helpful to check in with other parts of the body while you're in this pose. Notice if your shoulders, throat, and face are tense. If they are, relax them, and focus your awareness on grounding the left leg and breathing into the abdomen. Take 5 or more breaths before releasing the leg to the floor. Before practicing on the second side, take a moment to check in with your legs. Do they feel different from each other? If so, how?

FIGURE 30.
RECLINING LEG STRETCH POSE,
VARIATION

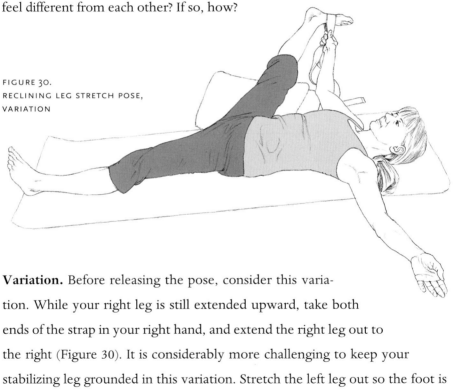

Variation. Before releasing the pose, consider this variation. While your right leg is still extended upward, take both ends of the strap in your right hand, and extend the right leg out to the right (Figure 30). It is considerably more challenging to keep your stabilizing leg grounded in this variation. Stretch the left leg out so the foot is pressing into the wall, as you stretch the right leg out to the right. I don't recommend letting the right leg rest on the floor, even if you are flexible enough to do so. When the leg rests on the floor, you lose the dynamic quality of the stretch. Instead, imagine lengthening both legs by extending the bones of both legs outward from the hips to the feet. That said, you may rest your outer, upper thigh on a folded blanket if you find yourself straining to hold your leg up. Stay for 5 or more breaths. Lift the right leg back up to vertical, and then lower the leg to the floor. Rest for a few breaths before moving to your second side.

Seated Angle Pose

UPAVISTHA KONASANA

▼ ▼ ▼ ▼ ▼ ▼ ▼ STRETCHES THE LEGS, HIPS, KNEES,
AND ANKLES • CALMS AGITATION

PRACTICE WITH CARE: If you have a diagnosed disc disease, do not bend forward in this pose.

PROPS: 1 nonskid mat • 1 or more blankets or a chair • 1 or 2 blocks

Nothing feels better for my legs after a long period of sitting in meditation than to stretch them out wide. While there are many wonderful forward bends in asana practice, Seated Angle Pose (Figure 31) hits the just the right note for hips, knees, and ankles that have been folded for a long time. In general, forward bends soothe agitation and help you contain energy, so this pose is appropriate when you're experiencing "monkey mind."

Sit on your mat with your legs spread to the sides at a 90-degree angle to each other. Now feel your lower spine. If you are feeling the lumbar spine poking out in back, this means that the lumbar is in flexion and your sacrum is not in its optimum angle. I don't recommend bending forward if your pelvis is tilting backward when you are in an upright sitting position. If this is the case, you will not be able to bend from the pelvis, but rather your spine will bend at the

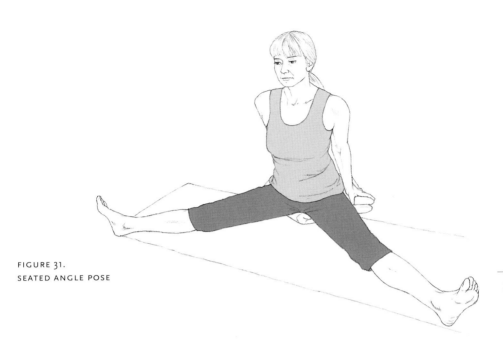

FIGURE 31.
SEATED ANGLE POSE

lumbar, which may put your discs at risk. Sit on one or more folded blankets, stacked so they are 4 to 8 inches high. If your pelvis is still tilting backward, place your hands behind you on the floor or on your blankets, and press into the floor with your fingers to bring your spine to an upright position. Now stretch out through the legs, and ground the backs of the thighs, calves, and heels on the floor. Take 5 or more deep breaths. To come out of the pose, bring your legs together so they are parallel to one another and rest here for a few breaths.

Variation. If you are able to bend forward from the pelvis and keep your spine in its natural curves—either with or without blankets—you can add a forward bend to this pose (Figure 32). Begin by grounding through the legs and lengthening them out to the sides. On an exhalation, begin walking your hands for-

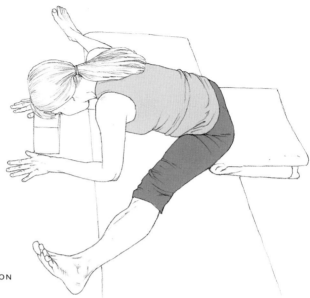

FIGURE 32.
SEATED ANGLE POSE, VARIATION

ward on the floor, allowing your abdomen and spine to lengthen as you move forward. Continuing to stretch out through the legs, let your body settle into whatever angle your inner thighs and hamstrings will allow. Relax your shoulders, neck, and facial muscles, and take 5 or more relaxing breaths.

It is particularly calming to the mind to rest your forehead on something in this pose. Since resting the forehead on the floor is not an option for most people, blocks and chairs can create the same effect for people of varying levels of flexibility. Place a block in front of you, or stack a couple of blocks, and let your forehead rest on them. You may also use the edge of a chair seat to rest your head. Even if you are very flexible, resting the forehead on a higher surface, such as a block or chair seat, can make Seated Angle Pose a lovely, settling experience.

Cannoli Roll

▼ ▼ ▼ ▼ ▼ ▼ ▼ RELAXES SHOULDERS AND NECK
QUIETS THE NERVOUS SYSTEM

PRACTICE WITH CARE: Lying on your back is contraindicated in the second and third trimesters of pregnancy.

PROPS: 1 nonskid mat • 2 blankets

Our shoulders and arms are our instruments of doing. We quite literally carry the weight of our daily lives on our shoulders. On long retreats, my experience of shoulder pain has given me some interesting insights about the nature of uncomfortable sensation. Even so, I'm all for doing whatever I can to soften the experience. The three poses in this "Softening the Shoulders" section have been helpful for me.

I learned Cannoli Roll (Figure 33) from Jenny Otto, a certified senior Anusara Yoga teacher and teacher trainer. Once you've set up in this wonderful restorative pose, you can stay as long as you want—10 or more minutes can bring about deep relaxation. This is a great pose to practice just before you climb into bed.

Begin by folding your blankets in quarters. Stack one on top of the other, so the long side of the blankets is facing you (in computer lingo, you are looking

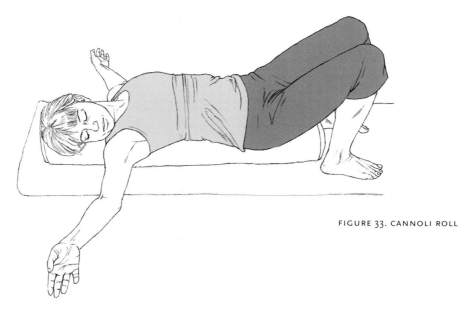

FIGURE 33. CANNOLI ROLL

at a "landscape" rather than a "portrait" orientation). Starting from that edge, roll the blankets up together, smoothing out wrinkles as you go. Take your time, and make sure the blankets are rolled firmly but not tightly together so the surface remains soft and the top surface is smooth.

Place your roll lengthwise on your mat. Sit on the end of the roll, with the rest of it behind you. Then lie down on the roll so your entire torso, from your tailbone to the top of your head, is supported. Let your arms relax out to the sides at about a 45-degree angle, and turn your palms up. Yield your weight completely to gravity, and breathe slowly and deeply, without straining or grabbing at the breath.

After a few minutes, slide your shoulders and arms 1 or 2 inches to the right, so your head rolls over to the right side. As you slide to the right, gently stretch your left arm out to the left. The inner border of your left shoulder blade will catch on the edge of your blanket, and you will likely feel a gentle stretch on the left side of your neck. Relax completely, allowing gravity to do the work for you. Continue long, luxurious breathing. After 1 or 2 minutes, slide your shoulders and arms back to the center, allowing your head to come up last. Relax in the center for 1 or 2 minutes before sliding the shoulders to the left for your second side. When you have finished your second side, return to the center and spend 1 or 2 minutes breathing and relaxing in the center. When you are ready to leave the pose, roll off your blankets onto either side, and take a few breaths here before pushing yourself up to sitting.

Supported Bridge Pose

SETU BANDHASANA

▼ ▼ ▼ ▼ ▼ ▼ ▼ ALLEVIATES NECK AND SHOULDER PAIN
EASES HEADACHES AND NERVOUS STRESS

PRACTICE WITH CARE: Do not practice this pose during your menstrual period or if you are pregnant. Avoid practicing backbends if you have spondylolisthesis or spondylolysis.

PROPS: 1 nonskid mat • 1 or 2 blocks • 2 straps (1 optional)
hand towel (optional) • athletic-type elastic bandage (optional)

Supported Bridge Pose (Figure 34) purifies the body as it calms the mind. Physically, the head-down position, combined with neck flexion, soaks the lymph glands in the neck and throat with blood. It also suppresses the fight-or-flight (sympathetic) side of the autonomic nervous system, restoring energy and supporting healing. When your head is below your heart and your neck is flexed, the baroreflex (a homeostatic mechanism for maintaining healthy blood pressure) is activated, setting off a chain of events that suppresses the sympathetic nervous system. This helps calm the mind for meditation. I've also found Supported Bridge Pose to be helpful in alleviating neck and shoulder discomfort that sometimes arises in meditation.

You can use an eye wrap in Supported Bridge Pose (see page 90). If you do, wrap it around your head before you lie down, but fold up the edge so you can see as you set yourself up. When you have moved into the pose with your hips on top of the block, carefully unfold your eye wrap so your eyes are gently covered.

Begin by lying on your mat with your knees bent and the soles of your feet on the floor, directly under your knees. Your feet should be hip-width apart. Press your feet into the floor to lift the hips up off the floor. Pick up your block and place it under your pelvis widthwise, so the entire sacroiliac joint is supported. Let your pelvis settle onto the block. If the block feels harsh under your pelvis, you can place a small folded hand towel on top to soften it.

The block has three potential heights, so feel free to experiment with orienting it the best way for your own spinal flexibility. You can stand it on its end if your hips lift pretty high off the floor, or you can place it on its side or flat on the floor if this feels better for you. In any case, make sure that your low back is not feeling strained. If it is, lower the block so your spine is at a less extreme angle.

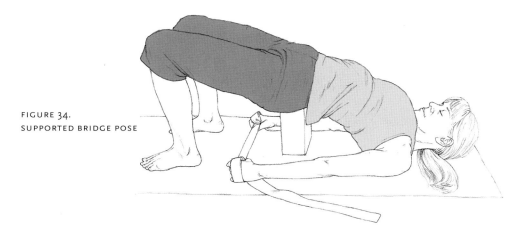

FIGURE 34.
SUPPORTED BRIDGE POSE

If your knees are uncomfortable in this position, try placing the narrow sides of a block between your knees and press gently into it. If this doesn't alleviate knee discomfort, try tying a strap around your thighs just above the knees, so the knees are hip-width apart. Then press gently out into the strap, as if you're going to stretch it.

Roll your shoulders under you, so your chest is expanding toward your chin. You can clasp your hands if they are able to reach each other. If you are unable to straighten your arms when your hands are clasped, use a second strap or belt to connect them, shoulder-width apart. Lengthen the front of your neck. Make sure your knees are still about hip-width apart. Now close your eyes, relax, and breathe slowly and deeply. You can stay in this pose for several minutes.

When you are ready to come out, lift your hips up off your block, and set the block aside with your hips still elevated. Stretch your arms out along the floor overhead, and slowly roll your spine down to the floor. When your hips reach the floor, move your arms to about a 45-degree angle next to your body and relax. After a few breaths on your back, roll onto your side, rest on your side for a few breaths, and then push yourself up to a sitting position. If you are using an eye wrap, fold it up to uncover your eyes while you are lying on your side. You may remove the eye wrap once you are sitting.

Eagle Arms Pose

GARUDASANA

▼ ▼ ▼ ▼ ▼ ▼ ▼ STRETCHES SHOULDER MUSCLES
OPENS THE UPPER BACK

PRACTICE WITH CARE: Practice gently and mindfully if you have shoulder, upper back, or neck problems.

PROPS: 1 nonskid mat • 1 strap • a zafu, v-shaped cushion, or meditation bench

The area between the shoulder blades can feel pretty cranky during sitting meditation. Expanding the chest, as in Cannoli Roll (Figure 33) and Supported Bridge Pose (Figure 34), can go a long way toward relieving shoulder stress. But sometimes stretching these muscles directly is the way to go. To do so, we'll practice the upper body part of Eagle Pose (Figure 14), which I call Eagle Arms Pose (Figure 35).

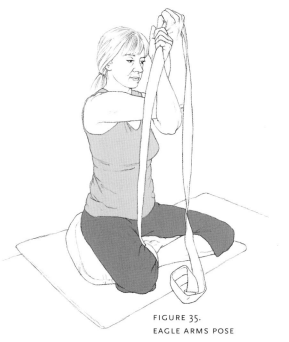

FIGURE 35.
EAGLE ARMS POSE

To begin, stand on your mat in Mountain Pose (Figure 12). Cross the right upper arm over the left, and place the fingers of your left hand into the palm of your right hand. If your fingers don't reach the right palm, use a strap to connect your hands. Direct your breath into the area between your shoulder blades. Take 5 to 10 breaths. Come back to Mountain Pose, and check in with your shoulders. How do your shoulders and upper back feel? Repeat on the other side.

You can practice Eagle Arms Pose from a variety of positions, including while seated. I often practice it while I'm sitting on my meditation cushion, both before I settle into my sitting practice and after I have finished. I have also practiced Extended Triangle Pose (Figure 18) and Extended Side-Angle Pose (Figure 20) with my arms in this position instead of with arms extended. Doing this places considerably more demand on your legs, which can be both invigorating for your legs and relaxing for your shoulders.

Revolved Belly Pose
JATHARA PARIVARTANASANA

▼ ▼ ▼ ▼ ▼ ▼ ▼ EASES BACK TENSION
CALMS THE NERVOUS SYSTEM

PRACTICE WITH CARE: Take it easy in this pose if you have diagnosed disc disease or if you are pregnant. In either case, stay well inside the limits of your ability to twist. If you have discomfort in your sacroiliac joint, place a folded blanket under your knees to raise them.

PROPS: 1 nonskid mat • 1 blanket

There's nothing like a gentle spinal twist to unravel tension in your back. Revolved Belly Pose (Figure 36) helps soothe complaining back muscles,

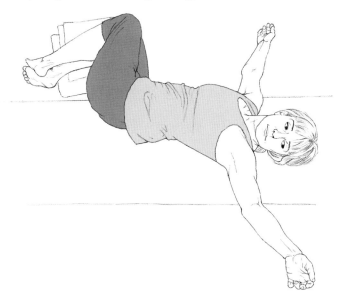

FIGURE 36.
REVOLVED BELLY POSE

whether you've been sitting at a desk or on a meditation cushion. It also massages your internal organs. Make sure to take advantage of your revolved abdomen in this pose by breathing very deeply to assist the natural massage of your vital organs. Revolved Belly Pose can help smooth out nervous agitation in your meditation practice.

Lie on your back on your mat, with your knees bent and the soles of your feet on the floor. Extend your arms out 90 degrees at shoulder level, and turn your palms upward. Draw both knees in toward your torso, so your thighbones are vertical. If you feel your buttocks starting to lift off the floor and your low back pressing into the floor, let your knees move away from your torso until your pelvis is again relaxed on the floor. Release your knees over to the right side, resting them on the floor. If you feel discomfort in your sacroiliac area, elevate your knees on a folded blanket while in the twist.

Do not attempt to align your left knee directly over your right. Instead, rest it on the right inner thigh, a few inches from your right knee. Turn your head to the left. Take 5 or more long, relaxing breaths. Lift your knees back up to vertical, and release your feet back to the floor. Take a few breaths in the center before moving to your second side.

If you experience neck discomfort in sitting meditation (or at other times) you might enjoy this variation: While you are in the pose, roll your head from side to side, very slowly and mindfully. Do not swivel the head like an owl, but rather roll in an arc, so that as you reach extreme right and left, your nose is pointing at your shoulder. Move very slowly, exploring the contours of your skull against the mat as your head rolls side to side.

Supported Bound-Angle Pose

SUPTA BADDHA KONASANA

▼ ▼ ▼ ▼ ▼ ▼ CALMS THE NERVOUS SYSTEM
SOOTHES THE DIGESTIVE SYSTEM • RELIEVES MENSTRUAL CRAMPS
OPENS THE INNER THIGHS • EASES MENTAL AGITATION

PRACTICE WITH CARE: If your knees or inner thighs feel uncomfortable in this pose, elevate your knees further with an additional blanket.

PROPS: 1 nonskid mat • 2 or 3 blankets

Supported Bound-Angle Pose (Figure 37) grounds "monkey mind" energy as it restores vitality. Its abdominal-opening quality focuses energy into the lower body, which in my experience can take the edge off mental agitation. Supported

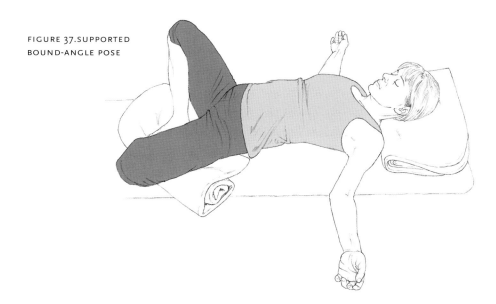

FIGURE 37. SUPPORTED
BOUND-ANGLE POSE

Bound-Angle Pose gently opens the inner thighs, making cross-legged sitting easier. It can also be helpful for digestive complaints and menstrual cramps. Since your body is completely supported, you need not exert effort to stay in the pose. Instead, allow yourself to let go of all effort and relax deeply.

Sitting on your mat, fold one of your blankets in quarters, and set it in front of you so the short side of the blanket is facing you. (It will be in "portrait" rather than "landscape" orientation as you look at it.) Fold your blanket over twice, so it is 8 to 10 inches wide. Set the blanket lengthwise on your mat behind you.

Now take your second blanket, set it in front of you, fold it in quarters, and then turn it, if necessary, so the long side faces you (in landscape orientation). Roll up the blanket from the long side so you have a long, snake-like roll. Bend your knees, place the soles of your feet together, and then draw the feet in close to your pubic bone. Place the center of your "snake" over both feet, and draw the ends underneath your shins and thighs, so your feet remain on the floor but the knees are supported to lift.

Lean back on your hands, lift your hips slightly off the floor, extend your tailbone down toward your heels, and then set your hips back down on the floor. Lie back on your first blanket, with your legs supported by the second one. Relax your arms onto the floor at about a 45-degree angle to your torso. If your head is tilting back, place another folded blanket or towel under your head and neck, so it barely grazes the tops of your shoulders. Feel free to add this head support even if your head is not tilting back.

Relax and breathe naturally into your abdomen. On your exhalations, let your body relax down into the floor as if you are gradually, with each breath, letting go of resistance to gravity. Allow your body to be completely supported.

Stay as long as you like, up to 20 minutes if you are comfortable. When you are ready to come out, lift both knees up to vertical, and gently roll onto either side. Stay on your side for a few breaths before pushing up to a sitting position.

Child's Pose

BALASANA

▼ ▼ ▼ ▼ ▼ ▼ ▼ SOOTHES INTERNAL ORGANS
EXPANDS THE BACK BODY • CALMS THE MIND

PRACTICE WITH CARE: If you have diagnosed disc disease, this pose may cause discomfort. If this is the case, separate your knees wider, so your torso relaxes in between them. If this does not relieve the issue, skip this pose for now. You can also widen your knees in Child's Pose to accommodate your growing belly if you are pregnant.

PROPS: 1 nonskid mat • 1 or more blankets • 1 hand towel

Child's Pose (Figure 38) evokes feelings of safety and comfort, as your body and mind turn inward. Practice it at any time during an asana sequence, especially when your mind and body feel agitated. Like Mountain Pose (Figure 12), it is a wonderful pose to come home to for regrouping, between other poses.

Begin by sitting on your heels on your mat. Separate your knees hip-width apart. On an exhalation, lean forward, letting your torso rest on your thighs. There are two options for your arms: You can rest your arms alongside your legs with your palms up or fold your arms on the floor in front of your head and turn your palms down. Whatever position you choose, relax your shoulder blades so they roll gently toward your head. Rest your forehead on the floor, or turn your head to one side if that is more comfortable. Remember to turn your head to the other side after a few breaths, so your neck stretches equally on each side.

If your knees are uncomfortable in Child's Pose, try placing one or more folded blankets on top of your calves and ankles, in the space between your lower legs and thighs. This changes the angle of the body and therefore the relationship of the head to the floor. You will likely want to place a folded hand towel under your head and turn your head to one side (turning it to the other side after a minute or so).

Child's Pose helps you develop awareness of your back body. We often focus our breathing in the front body, but because the lungs actually rotate outward and forward on the inhalation, Child's Pose supports the natural movement of your lungs. Take advantage of this by breathing deeply into your back body, allowing it to expand in all directions—vertically along the spine, horizontally, and in its circumference. Stay for up to 1 minute, breathing deeply and easily, creating space in your back body on your inhalation and settling into that space on your exhalation.

When you are ready to come out of the pose, gently ground your sitting bones and begin to roll the spine toward vertical from the bottom up, letting your head lift last. Take a few breaths and rest while sitting upright on your heels.

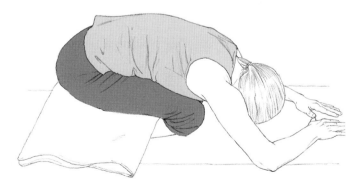

FIGURE 38. CHILD'S POSE

Eye Wrap

▼ ▼ ▼ ▼ ▼ ▼ ▼ RELIEVES EYE STRAIN
CALMS THE NERVOUS SYSTEM

PRACTICE WITH CARE: Set up each pose with your head wrap in place but with the front bottom edge folded up so your eyes are exposed. That way you can see until you have your body and all your props in place. Eye wraps obscure more light than your eyelids do on their own. Make sure to give your eyes time to adjust to the light after you remove your eye wrap.

PROP: 1 athletic bandage, about 3 inches wide • 1 nonskid mat or a chair

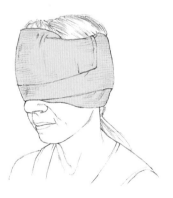

FIGURE 39. EYE WRAP

Wrapping your eyes and head while you practice asana is a nice option when you are feeling stressed or agitated. Unlike an eye pillow, an Eye Wrap (Figure 39) will not fall off, so you can use it in many poses. Try using it when you practice seated and reclining poses (but it's best not to use it in standing poses unless your balance is very steady).

To wrap your eyes, sit on your mat or chair. Start with your bandage rolled up. Take the loose end of the bandage and place it on the left side of your head if you are right-handed or on the right side of your head if you are left-handed. At this point, the bottom edge of the bandage should be just above your ear. Then begin wrapping the bandage loosely around your head, but tightly enough so you feel gentle contact with your forehead and eye sockets. Do not cover your nostrils. When you come to the end of the bandage, tuck the loose end into the wrap. Position your bandage so the loose end is not at the back of your head, creating an uncomfortable lump. If you need to see at any time during your practice, simply fold up the bottom of the bandage so your eyes are uncovered.

To remove your wrap, unravel it, rolling it back into a roll as you go so it is ready for the next time.

Basic Relaxation Pose
SAVASANA

▼ ▼ ▼ ▼ ▼ ▼ ▼ RELEASES TENSION
INTEGRATES ENERGIES

PRACTICE WITH CARE: Do not lie on your back after the first trimester of pregnancy; instead practice Side-Lying Relaxation Pose (on your left side, Figure 42.)

PROPS: 1 nonskid mat • 1 to 4 blankets
1 athletic bandage or eye pillow (optional) • 1 chair (optional)

In the mid-1980s, my mother and my aunt Charlotte attended a yoga for seniors class in Cincinnati. As an incipient yoga teacher in those days, I enjoyed listening to my mother and aunt talk about their class and how their teacher approached teaching yoga to people in their 60s, 70s, and 80s. My mother's and aunt's favorite pose was one their teacher called the Sponge.

As it turned out, the Sponge was what I called Basic Relaxation Pose (Figure 40). It is the pose that ends every asana practice. Back then I thought that the Sponge was a silly name for such a tranquil and profound pose, but as I practiced I realized that it's actually a helpful, descriptive image for this most essential pose. In Basic Relaxation Pose, your body soaks in the benefits of the asanas you've practiced, in the same way that water soaks into a sponge.

Basic Relaxation Pose is the most important of all the asanas. In this pose, we absorb and integrate the energies we've awakened in our practice. It is Basic Relaxation Pose that yields the lovely "transparent" feeling in your body after you finish your practice. It's what gives you the quiet glow that helps you move more gracefully through your day.

When we practice asana, breathing deeply as we slowly and gently stretch muscles and connective tissue, we stimulate circulation, maximize respiration, and set the stage for deep relaxation. When we lie in Basic Relaxation Pose for 10 to 15 minutes or more, the physiological systems of the body are able to relax.

As a culture, we undervalue relaxation. Consequently, as yoga has become Westernized, we give Basic Relaxation Pose short shrift when compared to more active poses. We Westerners consider doing to be more important than being. In reality, neither is more important than the other, but when we emphasize one over the other or, at the most extreme, practice one to the exclusion of the other, our lives move out of balance.

In using yoga practice as a tool to support meditation, Basic Relaxation Pose is essential. The pose is the essence of being. In Basic Relaxation Pose, you allow your body to be completely supported and receptive. As thoughts move

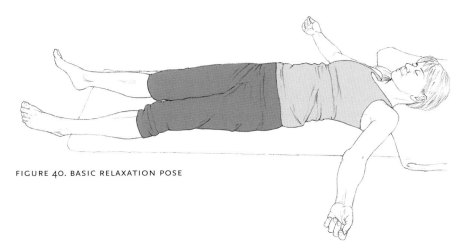

FIGURE 40. BASIC RELAXATION POSE

through your consciousness, there's nothing you need to do with them. Neither indulge them nor push them away. Just allow thoughts and sensations to roll on through your awareness, as if you're settling back and letting them pass by on a screen in front of you.

Spread your mat out on the floor. For more comfort, spread a blanket over your mat so it covers the entire length. If you would like to use an eye wrap, this is a good time to wrap it around your head. If you prefer, you may use an eye pillow instead. Lie on your back on your mat with your arms at about a 45-degree angle to your sides and your palms facing up. Extend your legs out about hip-width apart, and let them rotate naturally outward.

You can place a folded blanket under your head for support, especially if your head is tilting back. If you choose to use head support, place it under both your head and neck, so the edge of it barely grazes the tops of your shoulders. If your back is uncomfortable, place a rolled blanket under your knees to elevate them.

Now relax your breathing, and as you exhale, settle into the force of gravity. Breathe naturally and easily. Let your body breathe itself. Let awareness spread throughout your body, so it inhabits all your cells. Feel the gentle wave of the breath as it ripples through your tissues. Be aware of all the parts of the breath: inhalation, exhalation, and the still space between breaths. Explore and become familiar with the still point between your breaths; this is a place of pure being that is accessible to you at any time.

Stay in Basic Relaxation Pose for a minimum of 10 minutes, preferably 15 to 20 minutes. When you are ready to come out, begin breathing more deeply and intentionally. Take several breaths before beginning to move your hands and feet, opening and closing your hands, and flexing and extending the feet and ankles. When you are ready, bend your knees and place the soles of your feet on the floor. Roll completely onto one side, and rest here for a few breaths before using your top arm to assist you up to a sitting pose.

Relaxation Pose, with Calves on a Chair. If your back is still uncomfortable even with a blanket roll, practice with your calves on a chair (Figure 41). Position the chair close enough to your body so your thighs are vertical. After 10 to 20 minutes, draw your knees in toward your chest, and roll onto either side, resting there for a few breaths before using your top arm to push you up to a sitting pose.

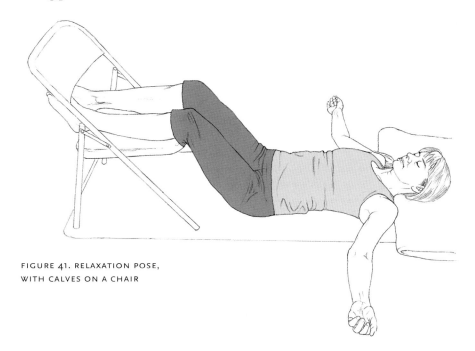

FIGURE 41. RELAXATION POSE,
WITH CALVES ON A CHAIR

Side-Lying Relaxation Pose. Place a blanket over your mat. Have three additional blankets handy, one folded so it is 5 or 6 inches thick, the second one folded to about 4 inches thick, and the third one rolled into a thick roll. The first blanket goes under your head and neck, like a pillow. Place the second folded blanket between your thighs and knees. Then place the third rolled blanket in front of you on the floor. Extend your bottom arm out at shoulder level underneath the roll, and drape your top arm over it. Draw the roll in so it extends along the length of your front body (Figure 42). Stay for 10 to 20 minutes. To come out, simply push yourself up to sitting using your top arm.

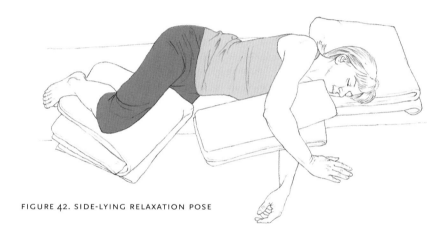

FIGURE 42. SIDE-LYING RELAXATION POSE

Part 3

Practicing Yoga

▼ ▼ ▼ ▼ ▼ ▼ ▼ ▼ ▼ ▼ ▼ ▼

FAQ

Should I consult with my doctor before doing yoga? Yoga practice is meant to heal and restore our energy. Even so, some poses may exacerbate chronic conditions such as high blood pressure, structural imbalances such as disc or joint issues, headaches, or menstrual and digestive issues. It's wise to talk to your doctor before embarking on any physical program.

How can I practice with care? Each pose description in part 2 begins with a synopsis of cautions, or ways to work with specific physical issues. If any of the poses presented in part 2 cause pain or discomfort, first try backing off and practicing more gently. If you still experience pain or discomfort, come out of the pose. Yoga should not hurt. Poses that cause you pain are probably not appropriate for you at this time.

If you are ill, practice lying down and supported poses such as Cannoli Roll, Revolved Belly, Supported Bridge, Supported Bound-Angle, Child's Pose, and

Basic Relaxation Pose. If you are injured, avoid poses that directly stress the area of injury. If a pose increases discomfort in an injured area, stop immediately.

During the active bleeding phase of menses, avoid standing poses, back bends, and any pose that places your hips above your heart, such as Supported Bridge Pose. Forward bends such as Pigeon Pose, Cross-Leg Revolved Pose, and Seated Angle Pose can be very helpful during menses. Supported Bound-Angle Pose can be especially helpful in alleviating menstrual cramps.

What are the benefits of going to class and of practicing on my own? Home practice is the cornerstone of a committed yoga or meditation practice. This book is designed to help you tailor a yoga practice to support your unique needs. That said, it is sometimes helpful to work with an experienced teacher who can help you find optimum alignment and give suggestions on how to use props to help you achieve the most easeful pose possible. An experienced teacher can see misalignments that we can't, and often a minor adjustment in a pose can open up a whole new world.

How often should I do yoga? Practicing yoga every day is ideal, but busy schedules can sometimes make a full daily yoga practice impossible. I like to qualify the suggestion to practice daily by encouraging you to commit to a small amount of time that you know you can keep to. It can be as little as 5 minutes or as long as 2 hours. What matters is that you do a little each day. You might try committing to short sessions on workdays and longer sessions on the weekends. It's important that you commit to a schedule that is doable for you. One pose a day is more beneficial than none!

Where is the best place and time of day to do yoga? How best can I work it in with meditation practice or during retreat? Find a quiet spot, away from others, undisturbed by television or the phone, so your mind can focus fully on what you are doing. If there's no such place in your home, do the best you can to anchor your mind to the sensations you feel in your body. Ask your family to grant you some quiet time. Practice is regenerative. When you replenish yourself, you have more energy to share.

I like to practice in the morning, because it sets a relaxed tone for my day and there are usually fewer distractions. But practicing in the evening, especially forward bends and lying down poses, can set you up nicely for evening meditation and sleep.

I particularly like to practice yoga asana before my sitting meditation practice, morning or evening. It relaxes my body and settles my mind so my meditation is more easeful. During retreats, if there is no formal group practice in the schedule, I retreat to my own room to practice yoga.

Can I eat before practice? Avoid practicing yoga for at least 2 hours after eating a full meal. Your yoga asanas will not feel very good on a full stomach, and yoga on a full stomach can sometimes cause indigestion. A light snack an hour before practice is usually okay.

What should I wear? Wear loose, comfortable clothing that allows freedom of movement. You need not have an expensive yoga-specific outfit. For home practice, anything that feels comfortable will work. If you plan to attend a class, it can be helpful if you wear stretchy clothing with some form-fitting qualities so your teacher can more easily see how you are aligned. Again, an expensive outfit isn't necessary. A simple T-shirt and stretchy pants or shorts will do.

What yoga props do I need? Yoga props were originally developed by B.K.S. Iyengar, an Indian yoga master, during the twentieth century. Props are designed to help us practice with greater ease. Some, like nonskid mats, help us practice safely and provide general cushioning in any pose. Others, like blocks, straps, or blankets, can help less flexible people enjoy the benefits of performing a pose to its fullest extent without creating strain. Props can help us relax deeply in supported poses. Here's what I recommend having in your collection:

- 1 nonskid mat
- 2 firm blankets
- 1 or 2 yoga blocks
- 1 8-foot strap
- 1 athletic-type bandage or eye pillow

Sequences

The following sequences are designed to help you address specific challenges you might encounter in your meditation practice. Any asana practice will be supportive, but the poses listed are here are the ones I've found to be most helpful in specific situations. Be mindful of your experiences as you practice, and if you find that varying these sequences is more effective to your unique needs, please do so. Feel free to mix it up: Add or omit poses; do poses you know and like that aren't in this book. Stay true to your body-mind's particularities on a given day in a given period of your life. Most important, enjoy the poses.

The asanas below are arranged as sequences, so you can practice them in the listed order to create a balanced session. If you don't have time for a full practice, choose two or three from the list, and always end with Basic Relaxation Pose (or one of its variations).

Remember: Yoga is the settling of the mind into silence. Yoga is neither a performance nor a competition. If you find yourself struggling to "get somewhere" in your yoga practice, explore the notion of letting go of that struggle, and relax into where you are. There is no pose out there in the future that's better than the one you are practicing right now. When you are at ease in the present, you will uncover your intrinsic silent center. Once revealed, that center can be your companion on your meditation cushion as well as in your everyday life. Let your asana practice be a meditation.

For Calming Agitation

Try an Eye Wrap (page 90) in any of the nonstanding poses in this list, from One-Leg King Pigeon Pose through Basic Relaxation Pose (or a variation). You can practice Child's Pose (page 88) as listed or insert it where it feels appropriate.

 1. Mountain Pose (page 35)

 4. Wall Dog Pose (page 45)

 2. Tree Pose (page 39)

 5. Wide-Leg Standing Forward Bend Pose (page 48)

 3. Eagle Pose (page 41)

 6. One-Leg King Pigeon Pose (page 63)

7. Cross-Leg Revolved
Pose (page 65)

8. Reclining Leg Stretch
Pose (page 68)

9. Seated Angle Pose
(basic or variation)
(page 72)

10. Cannoli Roll
(page 75)

11. Revolved Belly Pose
(page 83)

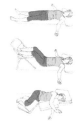

12. Supported Bound-
Angle Pose (page 85)

13. Child's Pose
(page 88)

14. Relaxation Pose
(basic or variations)
(pages 92, 95, 96)

For Increasing Energy

1. Mountain Pose

(page 35)

2. Tree Pose
(page 39)

3. Eagle Pose
(page 41)

4. Standing Side Bend

(page 43)

5. Wide-Leg Standing
Forward Bend Pose
(page 48)

6. Extended Triangle
Pose (page 50)

7. Warrior I Pose
(page 53)

 8. Extended Side-Angle
Pose (page 55)

 9. Lunge Pose,
Variation 1 (page 61)

 10. Lunge Pose,
Variation 2 (page 61)

 11. Lunge Pose,
Variation 3 (page 62)

 12. Supported Bridge
Pose (page 78)

 13. Revolved Belly Pose
(page 83)

 14. Seated Angle Pose
(page 72)

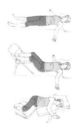 15. Relaxation Pose
(basic or variations)
(pages 92, 95, 96)

For Opening the Hips

 1. Mountain Pose
(page 35)

 2. Standing Side Bend
(page 43)

 3. Wide-Leg Standing
Forward Bend Pose
(page 48)

 4. Extended Triangle
Pose (page 50)

 5. Warrior I Pose
(page 53)

 6. Extended
Side-Angle Pose
(page 55)

7. Gate Latch Pose
(page 57)

 8. Lunge Pose,
Variation 1 (page 61)

 9. Lunge Pose,
Variation 2 (page 61)

 10. One-Leg King
Pigeon Pose
(page 63)

 11. Reclining Leg
Stretch Pose
(page 68)

 12. Supported Bound-
Angle Pose (page 85)

 13. Seated Angle Pose
(page 72)

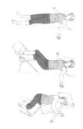 14. Relaxation Pose
(basic or variations)
(pages 92, 95, 96)

For Relieving Stress

Use an Eye Wrap (page 90), if you like, for all the seated and lying poses in this sequence. Stay several minutes in the last five poses and as long as 20 minutes in Relaxation Pose (basic or variations), if possible.

 1. Mountain Pose
(page 35)

 2. Standing Side Bend
(page 43)

 3. Wall Dog Pose
(page 45)

 4. One-Leg King Pigeon
Pose (page 63)

5. Cross-Leg Revolved Pose (page 65)

 6. Eagle Arms Pose (page 81)

 7. Reclining Leg Stretch Pose (page 68)

 8. Seated Angle Pose (page 72)

 9. Cannoli Roll (page 75)

 10. Supported Bridge Pose (page 78)

 11. Revolved Belly Pose (page 83)

 12. Supported Bound-Angle Pose (page 85)

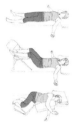 13. Basic Relaxation Pose (basic or variations) (pages 92, 95, 96)

FOR EASING THE LOWER BACK

A lot of poses can help the lower back, and you may not want to do all of these in a single practice. If your time is limited, choose one or more standing poses, a side bend, a back bend, a twist, and a forward bend. Finish with Relaxation Pose (basic or variations).

 1. Mountain Pose (page 35)

 2. Standing Side Bend (page 43)

 3. Wall Dog Pose (page 45)

 4. Wide-Leg Standing Forward Bend Pose (page 48)

5. Extended Triangle
   Pose (page 50)

6. Warrior I Pose
   (page 53)

7. Extended Side-Angle
   Pose (page 55)

8. Gate Latch Pose
   (page 57)

9. Lunge Pose,
   Variation 1 (page 61)

10. Lunge Pose,
    Variation 2 (page 61)

11. One-Leg King
    Pigeon Pose
    (page 63)

12. Cross-Leg Revolved
    Pose (page 65)

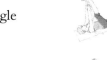

13. Reclining Leg Stretch
    Pose (page 68)

14. Seated Angle Pose
    (basic or variation)
    (pages 72, 74)

15. Supported Bridge
    Pose (page 78)

16. Revolved Belly Pose
    (page 83)

17. Supported Bound-
    Angle Pose (page 85)

18. Child's Pose
    (page 88)

19. Relaxation Pose
    (basic or variations)
    (pages 92, 95, 96)

For the Moon Cycle

Practice with care, and without force, during the active bleeding phase of your menstrual period. It's helpful to set an intention to practice in a relaxed way so you do not increase internal heat in your body. Let your period be a time of rest. Use an Eye Wrap (page 90) if you like.

 1. One-Leg King Pigeon Pose (page 63)

 5. Cannoli Roll (page 75)

 2. Cross-Leg Revolved Pose (page 65)

 6. Revolved Belly Pose (page 83)

 3. Reclining Leg Stretch Pose (page 68)

 7. Supported Bound-Angle Pose (page 85)

 4. Seated Angle Pose (basic or variation) (pages 72, 74)

 8. Child's Pose (page 88)

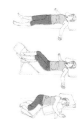 9. Relaxation Pose (basic or variations) (pages 92, 95, 96)

Feel free to explore any of the above sequences—all poses on each list, in order—as one long practice. Make sure you leave time for a 15-minute Relaxation Pose (basic or variation).

Part 4:

Alternate Meditation Postures

▼ ▼ ▼ ▼ ▼ ▼ ▼ ▼ ▼ ▼ ▼ ▼

Walking

I come from a family of walkers. The habit of walking was instilled in me at
an early age. On balmy evenings, spring through fall, my parents, sisters, and
I would walk the mile or so from our house to the Ohio River to watch the
ferryboat chug lazily over to the northern Kentucky shore, and to watch the
tugboats and barges glide downriver. My sisters and I always walked the mile
to school. My mother walked several miles a day well into her eighties. I've
always chosen to live in walkable neighborhoods. So when I began practicing
meditation, it was walking meditation that gave me my first access to the joys
of mindfulness.

Among its many attributes, walking meditation serves as a bridge between
sitting meditation and the rest of our daily lives. On vipassana (mindfulness, or
Insight Meditation) retreats, the alternation between sitting and walking meditation brings continuity to the practice. Soon, opening doors, eating, shower-
ing, washing dishes—all the activities of the day—become a meditation. I find

walking meditation to be the essential link that lifts meditation off the cushion and into the world.

In addition, walking meditation can bring a greater sense of energy and grounding to our lives. When I'm feeling dull and tired in my sitting practice, walking meditation can bring my energy up. When I'm nervous about something pending—maybe a solo I'm playing in a symphony—slow, mindful walking dissipates the agitation.

Taking a walk is not the same as walking meditation, even though any walk can be a mindful experience if that is the intention we bring to it. Walking meditation is a specific practice, designed to minimize the mental complications that can distract us from the actual experience of walking. In the absence of the decision of where to walk and how to walk, we are able to focus on the moment-to-moment sensations of walking.

There are many ways to practice walking meditation. For example, Zen walking, or *kinhin,* is different from what I offer here. The instructions that follow are based on the method I learned when I first began practicing Insight Meditation.

Begin by choosing a place for your walk. It may take you a few sessions to find the perfect place, but once you do, it is helpful to make that your designated path whenever you do your regular practice. You might want to choose a place outdoors for when the weather is cooperative and a place indoors for when it is not. Your own house and yard are fine places to practice.

Choose a path that is anywhere from 10 feet to 10 yards long. The distance doesn't really matter; in walking meditation, you do not walk to get somewhere. Choose a path with two clear endpoints. Then decide how long you will walk. It can be 5 minutes to an hour or more, depending on the time available to you. You practice walking meditation with shoes on, in your stocking feet, or barefoot, depending on where you walk.

In your meditation, you walk back and forth between your two chosen endpoints. Begin by walking at a pace slightly slower than your normal walking speed. Tune in your awareness to your legs and feet, and mentally note, "left, right, left, right" and so on, as each foot touches the ground. Walk at this speed for approximately a third of your walking period.

After you've walked at slightly slower than normal speed for the allotted time, slow down your pace. To give you an idea of the pace, it might take 10 seconds for you to take five or six steps, but this is by no means a precise or mandatory rate. Focus your awareness so you become conscious of the sensation of each heel, ball of your foot, and toes as they contact the ground. Mentally note, "heel, ball, toes" as you set your foot down. Keep this pace for another third of your walking period.

For the last third of your time, slow down even more, so you are walking very, very slowly. In this stage, be mindful of the sensations of lifting your foot off the floor, moving it through space, lowering it down, and setting the heel, ball, and toes onto the ground. Here you can mentally note, "lifting, moving, lowering, placing." Continue this slow, mindful walking until the end of your practice.

Depending on your unique propensities, you may fall into varying the practice in some way. For example, instead of precisely timing each third of the walking period, I've found that it is more natural for my walking to slow down gradually over time. Also, sometimes I want to start at a more brisk pace, and at other times, I start my walking pretty slowly. I let what feels right at a particular time dictate how I practice.

I find it important to honor whatever time commitment I've made for practice. So even if I'm feeling bored or tired, if I've committed to 20 or 30 minutes, I stick with it and allow my boredom or tiredness to be part of my mindfulness practice.

If you are away from your usual walking path for some reason, or you are visiting some beautiful or inspiring landscape, and you'd like to practice walking meditation, by all means, choose a couple of trees, rocks or other landmarks and make a walking path. Integrate the practice into your life in a way that works for you.

Yoga for Walking Meditation

When you begin practicing walking meditation, you will likely notice that the more slowly you walk, the more challenging it is to stay balanced. Microscopically slow walking is quite similar to balance exercises, because as one foot moves slowly through the air on its way to the ground, the other foot is supporting you entirely. So yoga poses that support balance are very helpful.

Although any of the poses in this book, practiced mindfully, are helpful, the poses I've found to be most specifically supportive of walking meditation are:

 1. Mountain Pose (page 35)

 2. Tree Pose (page 39)

 3. Eagle Pose (page 41)

 4. Extended Triangle Pose (page 50)

 5. Extended Side-Angle Pose (page 55)

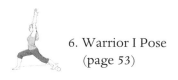 6. Warrior I Pose
(page 53)

 7. Wide-Leg Standing
Forward Bend Pose (page 48)

In addition, Reclining Leg Stretch Pose (page 68) and Seated Angle Pose (page 72) can help stretch leg muscles before and after walking.

You can also help increase your ability to balance by warming up your feet. Patsy, a septuagenarian student of mine who's been attending my classes since the 1980s, struggled with balancing poses for years. Then, in 2007, I learned some foot exercises from Jenny Otto and began teaching them in my classes. Patsy practiced these daily at home, and within six months she was able to balance on one leg away from the wall.

Foot Rejuvenating Exercises

FOOT MASSAGE

RESTORES TIRED FEET • STABILIZES BALANCE
IMPROVES CIRCULATION IN THE FEET AND LEGS

PRACTICE WITH CARE: Place a blanket under your hips if necessary to maintain your natural spinal curves. Alternatively, sit in a chair with both feet flat on the floor.

PROPS: 1 nonskid mat • 1 blanket • 1 tennis ball • a chair (optional)

Sit in Staff Pose (Dandasana) on your mat with your legs together and straight out in front of you. Place your left ankle across your right thigh. If you are sitting on the floor, you can bend your right knee and fold the leg into a cross-legged position underneath your left ankle if you like.

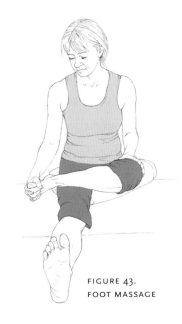

FIGURE 43.
FOOT MASSAGE

Thread the fingers of your right hand in between the toes of your left foot, interlacing them as deeply as you can into the webs between your toes (Figure 43). Then slowly and gently circle your ankle, 8 to 10 turns in each direction. With your fingers still between your toes, flex and extend the ball of your foot 8 to 10 times. Squeeze your fingers with your toes for a few breaths, and then squeeze your toes with your fingers for a few breaths. Remove your hand and massage your foot with both hands, from the toes through the ball and into the arch and heel. Take your time.

Then stretch both legs out (or return your left leg to chair-sitting position), and have a look at your feet. Notice if there's a difference in the appearance of your feet. Then repeat on the other side.

TENNIS BALL FOOT MASSAGE

RESTORES TIRED FEET • STABILIZES BALANCE
IIMPROVES CIRCULATION IN THE FEET AND LEGS

PRACTICE WITH CARE: If balancing on one foot is challenging for you, stand next to a wall so you can place one hand on the wall while you roll the tennis ball under your foot. You may also practice this while sitting in a chair.

PROPS: 1 nonskid mat or a chair • 1 tennis ball

Place a tennis ball on your mat, and stand in Mountain Pose (Figure 12) to the right of the ball. Place your left foot on the ball. Standing on your right foot, begin rolling the tennis ball under your left foot, massaging the toes, ball, arch, and heel with the ball (Figure 44).

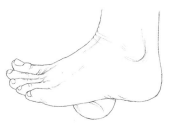

FIGURE 44. TENNIS BALL FOOT MASSAGE

Give the ball enough weight so you feel some pressure on the foot. Roll the ball under your foot for a minute or so, and then let it go. Stand in Mountain Pose, feeling not only the difference between the two feet but noting if you feel a difference between the right and left sides of your body. Repeat on the other side.

Lying Down

Of all the traditional meditation positions—sitting, walking, standing, and lying down—I've found lying down to be the most challenging. This may come as a surprise, as the idea of lying down sounds like quite a relief to many of us, including myself! But lying down and spacing out or falling asleep is one thing; lying down and maintaining an alert, mindful presence is quite another. Lying down and spacing out is the path of least resistance for most of us. Lying down signals rest time, and our body-mind habit is to drift off. Remaining awake and present while lying down requires some effort. I practice reclining when I am sick and when my energy is low. If I'm having trouble sleeping, I take advantage of my insomnia by practicing Lying Down Meditation. It relaxes my body and stills my mind so that even if I do not fall back to sleep, by meditating I'm restoring my body and mind.

Yoga for Lying Down Meditation. To practice, refer to the instructions for Basic Relaxation Pose (Figure 40) and its variations. You can meditate lying on your back with your legs stretched out straight on the floor, or you can prop the backs of your knees with a rolled blanket, or you can lie with your lower legs resting on the seat of a chair.

As in Basic Relaxation Pose, rest your mind on the breath in the body, either at a particular place, such as the nostrils or abdomen, or as a global awareness of the breathing body as a whole. Let your awareness enter all your cells, and feel the wave of your breath moving through your body. You can also bring awareness to the contact points between the body and the ground and how this relationship shifts as you inhale and exhale. This may help collect your awareness in a more concrete way.

Staying awake is a particular challenge in lying down meditation. You can help yourself stay more alert by setting yourself up in a supportive way. If you find you are drifting off, placing a folded blanket under your head and neck can be helpful. Also, when you are aware of yourself beginning to lose consciousness, bend one elbow and bring your forearm to upright. The energy required to keep your arm vertical may give you the lift you need to stay awake. If you tend to fall asleep in Lying Down Meditation, it can be helpful to practice with your eyes open, or with your eyelids just slightly closed.

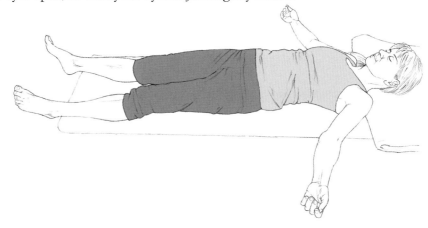

Yoga asanas help ease tensions in the body that can become uncomfortable when you stay still for a long period of time. Practicing any of the poses in this book will support ease and comfort in Lying Down Meditation.

Standing

Like Mountain Pose (Figure 12), standing meditation feels like coming home. I practice standing meditation on its own for its simultaneous energizing and calming effects, or in conjunction with sitting or walking meditation, particularly when I'm feeling out of balance.

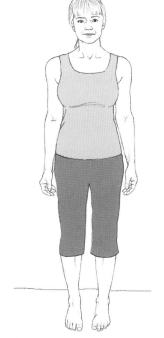

Standing meditation can neutralize your energies when you are feeling either sluggish or agitated. When I am sleepy in my sitting practice, getting up and standing can perk me up. The effort it takes to stand generates just enough energy to begin to dissipate the murky veil of sleepiness.

When I am feeling agitated in walking meditation and my mind is jumping all over the place, stopping and standing calms my energy. Sometimes when I am practicing walking meditation, I'll take the opportunity to practice standing meditation for a few breaths at each of the endpoints of my walking path. At other times, I stop in the middle of my path and stand for a period of time.

To practice standing meditation, refer to the instructions for Mountain Pose (page 35). Make sure your position is relaxed and self-supporting, with your spine in its natural curves. Let your breath be natural and easy. Be aware of the sensations of your feet connecting with the ground and your legs supporting you. Feel the entire body balanced over your legs, and tune in to the character of the energy in your body at this moment. Does it feel fast or slow, heavy or light, agitated or calm? Be present with what you feel in the body, especially the breath and the sensations in your feet and legs. Stay for a few minutes, up to 20 minutes or more if you can do so without strain. Do not practice standing for long periods if your blood pressure is low.

If I am practicing standing meditation outdoors, I sometimes combine it with hearing meditation. I simply stand and open my sense of hearing, allowing sounds to wash over me. Don't reach out for the sounds; simply allow them to come to you. They are coming anyway; there's no need to apply the extra effort of reaching for them. Instead, open the sense of hearing and allow your awareness to spread through your body, so you are hearing with your whole self, feeling the vibrations of sound in your body.

You can practice standing meditation anywhere—on its own as an intentional practice; in conjunction with sitting, walking, or hearing meditation; or even while you're standing in line at the bank or grocery store.

Yoga for Standing Meditation. The trick to standing in Mountain Pose for periods of time is to make sure, first of all, that the body is in a self-sustaining position. Review Setting Up (page 15), Active Yield (page 26), and Mountain Pose (page 35). All the poses described in this book will be helpful for standing meditation, but the poses that are particularly so are the same as those for walking meditation, including the Foot Massage (page 113) and Tennis Ball Foot Massage (page 114).

Resources

▼ ▼ ▼ ▼ ▼ ▼ ▼ ▼ ▼ ▼ ▼ ▼

YOGA WITH CHARLOTTE BELL

Charlotte Bell teaches ongoing classes in Salt Lake City. She also offers work-shops, retreats, and teacher trainings in Utah and surrounding states. For information about her schedule, visit her website at www.charlottebellyoga.com and on Facebook and Twitter (@MindfulYoga).

BOOKS

Charlotte Bell, *Mindful Yoga, Mindful Life: A Guide for Everyday Practice* (Berkeley, CA: Rodmell Press, 2007)

Donna Farhi, *The Breathing Book: Vitality and Health through Essential Breath Work* (New York: Owl Books, 1996)

Donna Farhi, *Yoga Mind, Body and Spirit* (New York: Owl Books, 2000)

Judith Hanson Lasater, Ph.D., P.T., *30 Essential Yoga Poses* (Berkeley, CA: Rodmell Press, 2005)

YOGA PROPS

Hugger Mugger Yoga Products
(800) 473-4888
www.huggermugger.com

ORGANIZATIONS

Insight Meditation Society
www.dharma.org

Spirit Rock Meditation Center
www.spiritrock.org

MEDITATION DVDs, CDs, AND DOWNLOADS

Dharma Seed
www.dharmaseed.org

About the Author

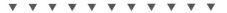

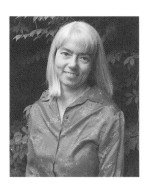

Charlotte Bell began practicing yoga in 1982 and began teaching in 1986. Guided by her teachers, Pujari and Abhilasha, founders of the Last Resort Retreat Center, in Duck Creek, Utah, she has blended the practice of yoga with that of Insight Meditation since 1986. She teaches workshops and retreats around the intermountain West and has served as faculty at several of Donna Farhi's international yoga teacher trainings in the United States and Canada. Each year, Charlotte teaches yoga on women's river rafting trips. She is currently board president for GreenTree Yoga, a nonprofit organization that brings yoga to underserved populations throughout Utah.

Charlotte is the author of *Mindful Yoga, Mindful Life*, published by Rodmell Press. She serves as a consultant for Hugger Mugger Yoga Products, and writes the blog on their website and a pose-of-the-month column for *Catalyst* magazine. She has modeled in asana photographs for Hugger Mugger Yoga Products catalogs and for *Yoga Journal, Yoga International,* and *Shambhala Sun* magazines.

A lifelong musician, Charlotte plays oboe and English horn with the Salt Lake Symphony and serves on their board of directors. She also performs regularly with the Scherzando Winds (a woodwind quintet), blue haiku (a chamber folk quartet), and Red Rock Rondo (a folk ensemble whose CD, *Zion Canyon Song Cycle*, has been released worldwide). In 2010 Red Rock Rondo's hour-long TV special won two Emmy Awards for best arts and entertainment special and best musical composition. The DVD also won a NETA (National Educational Television Association) Award for program production. Charlotte began writing feature articles for the Telluride Bluegrass Festival in 1991 and has been invited to collaborate on a book about the festival's thirty-five-year history.

Charlotte lives in Salt Lake City with her partner, Phillip Bimstein, and her three cats. Visit her website at www.charlottebellyoga.com and on Facebook and Twitter (@MindfulYoga).

From the Publisher

▼ ▼ ▼ ▼ ▼ ▼ ▼ ▼ ▼ ▼ ▼ ▼

Rodmell Press publishes books on yoga, Buddhism, aikido, and Taoism. In the Bhagavadgita it is written, "Yoga is skill in action." It is our hope that our books will help individuals develop a more skillful practice—one that brings peace to their daily lives and to the earth. We thank all those whose support, encouragement, and practical advice sustain us in our efforts.

CATALOG REQUEST

(510) 841-3123 or (800) 841-3123

(510) 841-3123 (fax)

info@rodmellpress.com

www.rodmellpress.com

TRADE SALES / UNITED STATES,
INTERNATIONAL

Publishers Group West

(800) 788-3123

(510) 528-5511 (sales fax)

info@pgw.com

www.pgw.com

FOREIGN LANGUAGE
AND BOOK CLUB RIGHTS

Linda Cogozzo, Publisher

(510) 841-3123

linda@rodmellpress.com

www.rodmellpress.com

Index

▼ ▼ ▼ ▼ ▼ ▼ ▼